Adjustment to Adult Hearing Loss

CONTRIBUTORS

Jack Ashley, M.A., Member of Parliament, Stoke-on-Trent, Staffordshire, England.

Pauline K. Ashley, M.A., M.Sc., Chairman, Committee of Management, Institute of Laryngology and Otology, London University, London, England.

Laurel E. Glass, Ph.D., Director, Center on Deafness, University of California, San Francisco, California.

Lesley G. Jones, M.Sc., Research Associate, Department of Mental Health and School of Education Research Unit, University of Bristol, Bristol, England.

Harriet Kaplan, Ph.D., Clinical Supervisor and Assistant Professor, Department of Audiology, Gallaudet College, Washington, D.C.

James G. Kyle, Ph.D., Research Fellow, School of Education Research Unit, University of Bristol, Bristol, England.

George L. Maddox, Jr., Ph.D., Professor of Sociology and Medical Sociology (Sociology and Psychiatry), and Chairman, University Council on Aging and Human Development, Duke University, Durham, North Carolina.

Kathryn P. Meadow-Orlans, Ph.D., Professor and Research Professor, and Director, Child Development Research Unit, Gallaudet College, Washington, D.C.

Harold Orlans, Ph.D., Consultant, Gallaudet Research Institute, and Special Assistant, U.S. Commission on Civil Rights, Washington, D.C.

E. Jane Oyer, Ph.D., Professor Emeritus, Department of Family and Child Ecology, Michigan State University, East Lansing, Michigan.

Herbert J. Oyer, Ph.D., Professor, Speech and Hearing Science, and Director, Department of Communication, Ohio State University, Columbus, Ohio.

Peter W. Ries, Ph.D., Chief, Illness and Disability Branch and Statistical Analyst, Health Interview Survey, National Center for Health Statistics, Washington, D.C.

Hilde S. Schlesinger, M.D., Professor in Residence, Department of Psychiatry, University of California, San Francisco, California.

Howard E. Stone, A.B., President and Director, Self-Help for Hard of Hearing People, Washington, D.C.

Peter L. Wood, B.A., Research Assistant, School of Education Research Unit, University of Bristol, Bristol, England.

Adjustment
to Adult
Hearing Loss

Edited by
Harold Orlans, Ph.D.

Gallaudet Research Institute
and U.S. Commission on Civil Rights

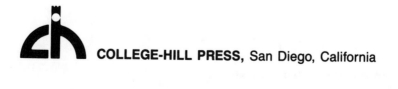

COLLEGE-HILL PRESS, San Diego, California

College-Hill Press, Inc.
4284 41st Street
San Diego, California 92105

Library of Congress Cataloging in Publication Data
Main entry under title:

Adjustment to adult hearing loss.

   Includes bibliographies and index.
   1. Aged, Deaf—Psychology—Addresses, essays,
lectures. 2. Deafness—Psychological aspects—Addresses,
essays, lectures. 3. Adjustment (Psychology)—Addresses,
essays, lectures. 4. Aging—Addresses,
essays, lectures. 5. Hearing aids—Addresses, essays,
lectures. I. Orlans, Harold, 1921-   [DNLM:
1. Hearing Disorders—in old age.   WV 270 A235]
HV2393.A35 1985   362.4'2'0880565   85-7761

ISBN 0-88744-180-7

Printed in the United States of America

CONTENTS

PREFACE

The chapters in this book were, with two exceptions, first prepared for and discussed at a monthly research seminar series on Hearing Loss in Adulthood sponsored by the Gallaudet Research Institute during the 1983-1984 academic year. One of the exceptions, the chapter by James Kyle and his associates, was included to fill a major gap in the literature dealing with the experience of persons who suffer a moderate hearing loss in midlife. The other, my own contribution, presents my observations and reiterates significant points made by a number of seminar members. Only after I had finished did I realize that these members, a distinct minority of the group, all happen to have had a profound hearing loss as adults; they *knew* what they were talking about.

The seminar arrangements illustrate what can be done to facilitate discussion among hearing, lipreading, and signing persons—and what can go wrong. A circle of two dozen chairs was surrounded by an audio loop; everyone—the chairman, speaker, and seminar members—used a microphone; and two interpreters, relieving each other in spells, translated speech to signs or signs to speech. The public lectures given by Hilde Schlesinger and Jack Ashley were complemented by a TV display of a stenotypist's transcript of the talk converted into readable text by a computer program, a system similar to the Palantype system Ashley has used to follow debates in the British House of Commons.

One long deafened professor was astonished at how much he heard with the loop. The arrangements usually worked well, although hearing-impaired persons undoubtedly lost some of the conversation. But at times the microphone did not work, spotlights shone in our eyes, and the clatter of dishes or noise of the air conditioner fan hampered hearing. The stenotype-TV demonstration required heroic efforts by a team of experts headed by Gallaudet's Donald Torr and court stenographer Martin Block; funny errors occurred when the program selected the wrong words for the right sounds. One speaker gave the interpreters trouble by talking too fast, though asked repeatedly to slow down; technical terms were also troublesome. However, the interpreters were an able and impressive group of young men and women.

Raymond J. Trybus, Dean of the Gallaudet Research Institute, authorized this project, chaired most sessions, invited and helped to select seminar members, and provided financial and administrative support throughout the two years from the start of planning to the completion of this book. He did so as a means of appraising the slight body of knowledge about adventitiously deafened persons and perhaps of stimulating research to improve knowledge about and the services for this large and relatively neglected population. Without his support, this book would not exist.

My wife, Kathryn Meadow-Orlans, who introduced me to the literature on deaf and hearing-impaired persons, has been a reliable, knowledgeable, and wise adviser at every stage of this project from the time it was merely an idea we talked about through the final corrections of references and proofs. No one could have a better adviser or wife.

Lucy Trivelli, assistant to Dean Trybus, ensured that all the seminar arrangements went smoothly; Sally O'Rourke, administrative assistant to the Dean, oversaw, and Carol Bennetti and Lola Wanner did all the typing and retyping of the manuscript.

Others who were helpful, especially during the initial discussions about prospective seminar topics, authors, and participants, included Peggy Williams of the American Speech-Language-Hearing Association; Howard Stone, founder of Self-Help for Hard of Hearing People; and Harriet Kaplan, James Pickett, and Teena Wax of Gallaudet College.

The members and guests of the seminar, who came from Gallaudet, other institutions in the Greater Washington area, and occasionally further afield, contributed much to its success. Subjecting the authors' ideas to the test of their own experience and knowledge, they engaged in a common search for enlightenment about the condition of hearing-impaired people, of which this book is a product.

Harold Orlans
Chevy Chase, Maryland

ACRONYMS AND ABBREVIATIONS

ANSI American National Standards Institute

ASA American Standards Association

ASL American Sign Language

COHI Consumers Organization for the Hearing Impaired

dB Decibel, a unit for measuring the relative loudness of sounds equal approximately to the smallest degree of loudness ordinarily detectable by the human ear, the range of which includes about 130 decibels on a scale beginning with 1 for the faintest audible sound (*Webster's Third New International Dictionary*)

FM A frequency modulation broadcasting system

HANES Health and Nutrition Examination Survey (same as NHANES), a national medical and health examination survey conducted by the National Center for Health Statistics

HES Health Examination Survey of the National Center for Health Statistics, expanded in later years into the HANES (also called NHANES)

HIS Health Interview Survey of the National Center for Health Statistics

Hz Hertz, a unit of frequency equal to one cycle per second

NCDP National Census of the Deaf Population, 1970-1972, directed by Jerome Schein and published in J.D. Schein and M.T. Delk, Jr. (1974). *The deaf population of the United States.* Silver Spring, MD: National Association of the Deaf

NCHS National Center for Health Statistics, Public Health Service, U.S. Department of Health and Human Services (formerly U.S. Department of Health, Education, and Welfare)

NHANES Same as HANES. National Health and Nutrition Examination Survey of the National Center for Health Statistics, a version of the Health Examination Survey expanded in 1971 to include nutrition

NHES Same as HES. National Health Examination Survey of the National Center for Health Statistics

NHIS Same as HIS. National Health Interview Survey of the National Center for Health Statistics

OUT Organization for the Use of the Telephone

Shhh Bimonthly journal of Self-Help for Hard of Hearing People

SHHH Self-Help for Hard of Hearing People, a voluntary national organization of hard-of-hearing people formed in 1979

TDD Telecommunication device for the deaf

TTY Teletypewriter, an electromechanical teleprinter

WAGHOH Washington Area Group for the Hard of Hearing

PART I

THE HEARING-IMPAIRED POPULATION

Chapter **1**
The Demography of Hearing Loss

Peter W. Ries

Anyone who prepares estimates of the number of persons with hearing trouble knows that there are no simple answers to such questions as how many people are deaf and how many individuals have serious trouble hearing. Since such estimates depend on how the degree of hearing loss is defined and the type of data used, it is as valuable to acquaint serious data users with the source of the estimates as with the estimates themselves. In this way, they may find the estimate that most closely matches their need and understand its limitations. Hence this chapter will start with a brief description of the major sources of estimates of hearing loss in the general population and the prevalences of hearing loss derived from them.

THE PREVALENCE OF HEARING IMPAIRMENT

Health Interview Survey Estimates

The National Health Interview Survey (NHIS) is an annual survey of about 40,000 households conducted by the National Center for Health Statistics. Bureau of the Census interviewers visit these households and ask a series of questions about the health and sociodemographic characteristics of each resident family member. Each year since, and periodically before, 1978 this survey yielded an estimate of the number of civilian noninstitutionalized persons with a hearing problem or tinnitus; these estimates were derived from responses to a three-part question: "Does anyone in the family now have (1) deafness in one or both ears, (2) any other trouble hearing with one or both ears, or (3) tinnitus or ringing in the ears?"

Most of the data presented in this paper have already been published in the cited sources. I would like to thank Michael Rowland of the National Health and Nutrition Examination Survey for preparing a few special tabulations from that survey.

The NHIS estimates indicate an overall increase in the prevalence and the prevalence rate of hearing trouble and tinnitus from 1971 to 1981 (Table 1-1), due solely to increases among persons under age 17 and 45 to 64 years old. In these estimates, the prevalence rate is more reliable than the prevalence frequency, since the Census Bureau underestimated the United States population during the 1970s, affecting the frequencies but probably not the rates shown in Table 1-1. The 1981 estimates are based on the 1980 decennial census, whereas those from 1977 to 1980 are based on the earlier underestimates.

The responses to these screening questions do not meaningfully distinguish the ability of people with various levels of hearing to function in the everyday world. To augment these data, every several years the NHIS adds a special supplement with a question on the use of a hearing aid and a short self-rating scale, the so-called Gallaudet Hearing Scale (Figure 1-1). This supplement is asked of all persons for whom deafness or trouble hearing (but not *only* tinnitus) was indicated in the screening questions. The responses permit classifying people by their unilateral or bilateral hearing loss and the degree to which they can hear and understand speech.

These hearing scale questions were included in the 1971 and 1977 surveys. Since these questions were not asked of persons who reported only tinnitus or children under age 3, the 14.2 million estimated number of persons with hearing problems in 1977 shown in Table 1-2 is smaller than the 16.2 million estimated number in Table 1-1. Nonetheless, the estimates in Table 1-2 are potentially far more useful than those in Table 1-1. For instance, they indicate that about half (7.2 million) of those with a hearing loss have a bilateral loss, the main concern of individuals and agencies in the field of deafness and hearing impairment.

Health Examination Survey Estimates

Another major source of estimates of hearing ability in the general population is the National Health Examination Survey (NHES). This survey, conducted in cycles since 1960, involves the clinical examination of representative national samples of specified age groups in the civilian noninstitutionalized population. After a household interview, respondents are asked to go to a specially constructed mobile examination unit where a doctor, nurses, dietician, and other professionals (including health technicians trained by audiologists) conduct examinations on many aspects of health and nutrition.

Table 1-3 summarizes the vast amount of data this survey has collected on the hearing ability of the United States population. Because each person undergoes many types of examinations, the health, nutritional (since 1971), and sociodemographic characteristics of persons with different hearing levels can be extensively described.

Table 1-1. Number of Persons with Hearing Impairments Including Tinnitus, and Number of Persons per 1,000 Population, by Age and Year, 1971 and 1977-1981, as Reported in Health Interview Survey: United States

Age	1981	1980	1979	1978	1977	1971
	Number in Thousands (by Year)					
All ages	18,666	17,370	16,663	16,540	16,219	14,491
Under 17	1,043	1,046	839	958	856	863
17-44	4,257	4,063	4,069	3,799	3,480	3,167
45-64	6,315	5,511	5,182	5,307	5,365	4,765
Over 64	7,051	6,750	6,573	6,477	6,518	5,695
	Number per 1,000 Population (by Year)					
All ages	82.9	79.7	77.2	77.4	76.4	71.6
Under 17	17.7	18.1	14.4	16.2	14.3	13.0
17-44	43.8	43.8	44.9	42.9	40.2	42.4
45-64	142.9	126.6	119.2	122.3	123.7	114.1
Over 64	283.8	282.5	281.6	284.2	292.7	294.3

Source: Feller (1977), Wilder (1978), and unpublished Health Interview Survey data.

HEARING SUPPLEMENT	R1	☐ No Hearing Problem (NP) ☐ A, B, or 33 in C2 (1-3)			
1. Has — ever used a hearing aid?	1.	1 Y 2 N			
(Hand Card H) Please look at this card — 2a. Which statement best describes —'s hearing in his *left* ear (without a hearing aid)?	2a.	Good 1☐	Little trouble 2☐	Lot of trouble 3☐	Deaf 4☐
b. Which statement best describes —'s hearing in his *right* ear (without a hearing aid)?	b.	Good 1☐	2☐	3☐	4☐
If age 3+, ask:	3a.	☐ Under 3 *(R2)*			
3a. (Without a hearing aid) Can — usually *hear and understand* what a person says without seeing his face if that person *whispers* to him from across a quiet room?		1 Y *(R2)* 2 N			
b. (Without a hearing aid) Can — usually *hear and understand* what a person says without seeing his face if that person *talks in a normal voice* to him from across a quiet room?	b.	1 Y *(R2)* 2 N			
c. (Without a hearing aid) Can — usually *hear and understand* what a person says without seeing his face if that person *shouts* to him from across a quiet room?	c.	1 Y *(R2)* 2 N			
d. (Without a hearing aid) Can — usually *hear and understand* a person if that person *speaks loudly* into his better ear?	d.	1 Y *(R2)* 2 N			
e. (Without a hearing aid) Can — usually tell the sound of speech from other sounds and noises?	e.	1 Y *(R2)* 2 N			
f. (Without a hearing aid) Can — usually tell one kind of noise from another?	f.	1 Y *(R2)* 2 N			
g. (Without a hearing aid) Can — hear loud noises?	g.	1 Y *(R2)* 2 N			

Figure 1-1. National Health Interview Survey questions asked of respondents who indicated hearing trouble, also known as the Gallaudet Hearing Scale.

Table 1-2.   Number of Hearing Impaired Persons 3 Years of Age and Over, by Hearing Ability, Level, and Type of Hearing Trouble, 1977

	Number (Thousands)
All persons 3 years and over	202,936
No hearing trouble	188,696
*Some hearing trouble**	14,240
Bilateral trouble†	7,208
At best, can hear words shouted in ear	842
Can hear words shouted across a room	2,310
Can hear words spoken in a normal voice	3,984
Unilateral hearing trouble	5,969
Hearing trouble borderline or unclear if unilateral or bilateral	985

* Includes 78,221 persons who did not respond to either hearing scale.
† Includes 71,144 persons who did not respond to the Gallaudet scale.
From Ries, P.W. (1982). Hearing ability of persons by sociodemographic and health characteristics: United States, (Series 10, No. 140). National Center for Health Statistics. Washington, DC: U.S. Government Printing Office.

Most of these audiological data have been reported in terms of the right or left ear hearing levels at specific frequencies. However, Table 1-4 presents the better-ear averages found in the first four survey cycles and the Committee on Conservation of Hearing's proposed classification of hearing impairments by the speech comprehension groups associated with different better-ear averages.

If a significant bilateral hearing loss is defined as a better-ear average of 26 dB or greater (American National Standards Institute, 1969), in the period 1974 to 1975 an estimated 8.7 million persons 25 to 74 years of age experienced, at best, difficulty only with faint speech; about 2.5 million with a better-ear average of 41 dB or more experienced "at best frequent difficulty with normal speech."

Neither of these estimates approximates the 1977 NHIS estimate of 4.7 million persons ages 25 to 74 with a bilateral hearing problem. Such differences are common in estimates obtained by radically different procedures.

Reconciling the Estimates

One way to reconcile the estimates is to examine the data from each survey and choose the better-ear average which produces approximately the same number of cases as the number with the bilateral hearing loss associated with responses to the hearing scale. A less simple, or simplistic, course is to administer both tests to the same population and determine the empirical relationship between the hearing levels identified by responses to the hearing

Table 1-3. Audiometric Data from National Examinations Surveys, by Years, Ages, Hertz Frequencies, and Number Sampled and Examined, 1960-1980

Survey	Years	Ages	Reference Zero	Air Conduction (Hz)	Bone Conduction (Hz)	Number Sampled/ Examined
HES I	1960-1962	18-74	ASA	500; 1000 2000; 3000 4000; 6000	No	7710/ 6672
HES II	1963-1965	6-11	ASA	250; 500 1000; 2000 3000; 4000 6000; 8000	No	7417/ 7119
HES III	1966-1970	12-17	ASA(82%) ANSI(18%)	250; 500 1000; 2000 3000; 4000 6000; 8000	No	7514/ 6768
NHANES I (Detailed sample)	1971-1974	25-74	ANSI	500; 1000 2000; 4000	500; 1000 2000; 4000	5593/ 3854
NHANES I (Augmentation)	1974-1975	25-74	ANSI	500; 1000 2000; 4000	No	4288/ 3059
NHANES II	1976-1980	4-19	ANSI	500; 1000 2000; 4000	No	7279/ 5901

HES, Health Examination Survey.
NHANES, National Health and Nutrition Examination Survey.
ASA, American Standards Association, 1951.
ANSI, American National Standards Institute, 1969.

scale and by audiometric examinations. This has been done on at least two occasions: in the mid-1960s, during the development of the Gallaudet Hearing Scale, when the scale and an audiometric examination were administered to a sample of 256 persons (age 18 and over) in the Philadelphia metropolitan area (Table 1-5); and in the period 1974 to 1975, when that scale and audiological examinations were administered by NHES to a sample of 3,059 persons ages 25 to 74 (Table 1-6).

The scale scores in Tables 1-5 and 1-6 represent the first question to which a "yes" response was given. For instance, a score of 3 means that the respondent could not hear and understand normal speech across a quiet room (question 2) but could hear and understand shouted speech across a quiet room (question 3). As may be noted in these tables, the mean better-ear average, in decibels, tends to rise markedly at each higher scale score. However, in both studies, so few persons with a scale score above 3 were interviewed that the associations are of little statistical significance. Hence these general population samples link hearing scale and audiological measures for persons with mild or moderate but not serious hearing losses. Thus, the problem persists of how to link these two sources of data meaningfully to produce a single estimate of the number of persons with a serious hearing loss.

Large sampling errors are a particular manifestation of the more general problem of obtaining representative and reliable data on persons with serious hearing trouble. One can obtain a sufficient number for detailed analyses from those who seek hearing services without knowing the prevalence of their hearing levels in the general population and the representativeness of the analyses, or one can determine prevalence from a general population survey but not have a sufficient number for reliable analyses of those with a serious hearing loss.

To solve this problem, the National Census of the Deaf Population (NCDP) used a three-phase research design. First, a large list of potentially deaf persons was constructed. The persons on this list were surveyed and those who were not deaf were excluded. Next, this revised list was computer-matched with the 1971 NHIS national sample, yielding a large number of persons with serious hearing trouble *and* a means of comparing them with persons of all hearing levels in the general population. In the final stage, extensive interviews were conducted with a relatively large representative sample of deaf persons extracted from the computer-matched list.

NCDP estimates of the number of persons with various types of hearing loss are given in Table 1-7. This census reported on a wide range of sociodemographic, educational, occupational, and health characteristics of the estimated 411,000 deaf persons who lost their hearing before the age of 19—the so-called "prevocational deaf." However, due to budgetary limitations, the NCDP did not conduct audiological examinations. A full

Table 1-4. Estimated Percentages of the Population with Various Hearing Levels

Mean Hearing Level in Decibels*		Speech Understanding	Ages and Years Surveyed†			
ASA	ANSI		18-79 1960-1962	6-11 1963-1965	12-17 1966-1970	25-74 1974-1975
Under 15 dB	Under 26 dB	Insignificant difficulty with faint speech	91.6	99.2	98.8	91.9
15-29 dB	26-40 dB	Difficulty only with faint speech	5.7	0.7	1.0	5.8
30-44 dB	41-55 dB	Frequent difficulty with normal speech	1.6	0.1	0.2	1.2
45-59 dB	56-70 dB	Frequent difficulty with loud speech				
60-79 dB	71-90 dB	Understands only shouted or amplified speech	1.1	—	—	1.1
Over 79 dB	Over 90 dB	Usually cannot understand even amplified speech				
All dB levels	All dB levels		100.0	100.0	100.0	100.0

ASA, American Standards Association, 1951; ANSI, American National Standards Institute, 1969.
* Re audiometric zero for 500, 1000, and 2000 Hertz in the better ear.
†The first three surveys were conducted by the Health Examination Survey and the fourth by the Health and Nutrition Examination Survey, as it was then renamed.
  Source: Glorig and Roberts (1965), Roberts and Haber (1970), Roberts and Ahuja (1975), and unpublished data for 1974-1975.

Table 1-5.   Number of Cases, Mean Better-Ear Hearing Level, and Standard Deviation, by Hearing Scale Score: Philadelphia Study, 1966 *

		Hearing Scale Score				
	Total	*1*	*2*	*3*	*4*	*5-8*
Number of cases	256	146	80	22	4	4
Mean better-ear hearing level in decibels†	19.1	13.2	19.5	44.4	41.3	64.5
Standard deviation		10.1	12.2	16.6	16.7	22.7

* Hearing scale was administered to a sample of 256 persons over 17 years old. The hearing scale score indicates number of first question to which respondent answered "yes"; see Figure 1-1 for questions used in the scale.

†Arithmetic average of hearing levels, in decibels, at 500, 1000, and 2000 cycles per second.

From Schein, J., Gentile, A., and Haase, K. W. (1970). *Development and evaluation of an expanded hearing loss scale questionnaire* (Series 2, No. 37). National Center for Health Statistics. Washington, DC: U.S. Government Printing Office.

range of audiological and hearing scale data has yet to be obtained for a large sample.

Nursing Home Data

The surveys considered so far are of the civilian noninstitutionalized population. The National Center for Health Statistics also periodically surveys a sample of nursing homes; data are obtained about the residents, recent discharges, and characteristics of the homes.

The data on the sample of residents, provided by knowledgeable persons in the nursing homes, classifies residents' hearing ability by responses to such categories as "(1) partially impaired—can hear most of the things a person says, (2) severely impaired—can hear only a few words a person says or loud noises, and (3) completely lost—deaf." In the most recent (1977) survey, 906,000 or 68 per cent of the estimated 1,330,000 nursing home residents were classified as not hearing impaired; 283,000 (21 per cent), as partially impaired; 56,000 (4 per cent), severely impaired; and 9,000 (1 per cent), deaf. About 49,000 could not be classified. As expected, the prevalence of hearing loss in this population is far greater than in the noninstitutionalized population.

Even this brief review of major sources of hearing loss estimates and prevalences should substantiate the initial statement that there are no simple answers to such questions as how many persons are deaf and how many have a serious hearing loss. Clearly, the answers depend on the definitions of the levels and types of loss and the methods for measuring them.

This discussion should promote skepticism about easy answers, but not pessimism about meaningful estimates of the magnitude of hearing loss

Table 1-6. Number of Persons 25-74, by Better-Ear Average Hearing Level for 500, 1000, and 2000 Hertz, Hearing Scale Score, and Standard Error of Mean: United States, 1974-1975

Hearing Scale Score*	Better-Ear Average in Decibels† of Persons 25-74 Years Old (in Thousands)									Standard Error of Mean
	All Levels	Less than 26	26 to 40	41 to 55	56 to 70	71 to 90	91 or more‡	Unknown	Mean‡	
All scores	108,494	99,023	6,204	1,330	685	387	111	753	11.1	0.41
1	85,413	81,638	2,956	141	35	83	—	559	8.9	0.32
2	19,691	16,356	2,473	487	197	37	—	141	15.5	0.70
3	2,854	894	704	659	381	164	—	53	37.2	2.77
4	301	100	44	43	43	71	—	—	43.0§	9.32§
6	26	—	26	—	—	—	—	—	27.0§	—§
7	41	—	—	—	29	—	12	—	77.3§	7.33§
8	132	—	—	—	—	33	99	—	96.0§	1.76§
Unknown	35	35	—	—	—	—	—	—	-7.0§	—§

— Data not available.

* Scaled index of hearing impairment based on questionnaire (see Figure 1-1); no response for scale score 5.

† Re audiometric zero, American National Standards Institute, 1969; excludes those with one or more missing hearing levels at 500, 1000, or 2000 Hz.

‡ All persons with hearing levels of 100 dB or more were coded "99"; the distribution of average hearing levels for 500, 1000, and 2000 Hz will reflect this truncation.

§ Data do not meet standards of reliability or precision.

Source: Unpublished HANES data.

Table 1-7. Prevalence and Rates (per 100,000 Population) of Hearing Impairments in the Civilian, Noninstitutionalized Population, by Degree of Impairment and Age at Onset, 1971

Degree of Impairment	Age at Onset	Number (Thousands)	Rate (per 100,000 Population)
Total hearing impairment	All ages	13,363	6,603
Significant bilateral	All ages	6,549	3,236
Deafness	All ages	1,767	873
	Under 19	411	203
	Under 3	202	100

From Schein, J., and Delk, M., Jr. (1974). *The deaf population of the United States.* Silver Spring, MD: National Association of the Deaf

in the general population. It is encouraging that, as has been shown, estimates are available on the number of persons within a given range of better-ear averages and the number who have difficulty hearing and understanding various levels of speech, and that a start has been made in determining the relation between these radically different ways of measuring hearing loss.

CHARACTERISTICS OF HEARING-IMPAIRED PERSONS

Without entering the controversy about whether there is a distinct deaf subculture, it is clear that hearing-impaired people are not a homogeneous group. The child in a residential school for the deaf and the deaf retired person face different problems, as do one retired person who was born deaf and another who recently lost his or her hearing. This section will examine several demographic features of the hearing-impaired population, starting with two of the most important: present age and age at the onset of hearing loss.

Hearing Loss and Age

The overwhelming association between increasing age and the increasing prevalence of hearing trouble is dramatically displayed in Figure 1-2, in which 1977 NHIS data are charted. An age chart of the hearing population resembles a pyramid; one of people with a hearing loss resembles an inverted pyramid, the shape differing only in degree for all those with a loss and those with a serious loss. Persons 70 years old and over make up 5.2 per cent of the hearing population but 30.2 per cent of the population with a hearing loss. Fully 49.3 per cent of those with a serious loss

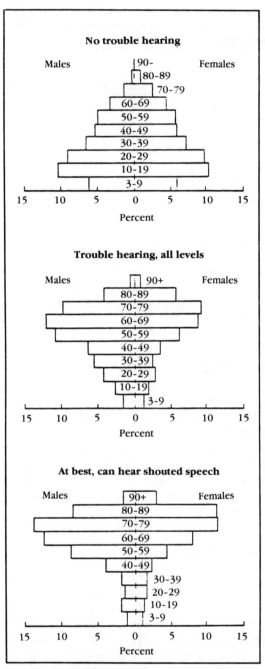

Figure 1-2.   Per cent distribution of persons 3 years of age and over, by sex and age, according to hearing ability. From Ries, P.W. (1982). *Hearing ability of persons by sociodemographic and health characteristics: United States.* (Series 10, No. 140). National Center for Health Statistics. Washington, DC: U.S. Government Printing Office.

(who can at best hear only shouted speech) are age 70 or over. The mean better-ear average rises from 5.4 dB for persons 25 to 34 years old to 21.9 dB for those 65 to 74 years of age (Table 1-8).

Knowledge of the age of onset of hearing loss is vital to the meaningful classification of hearing-impaired persons. Unfortunately, the 1977 NHIS did not determine age at onset and the NHANES, which did, has yet to tabulate these data.

However, the 1971 NHIS did contain a question about age at onset; Table 1-9 shows the relationship between degree of hearing loss, age, and age at onset of the loss. Twenty-four per cent of persons 3 years old or older with a serious hearing loss experienced the loss before the age of 21. Two thirds of those aged 17 to 44 but only a tenth of those over 64 had a hearing loss before 21. Thus, the prevocational deaf (defined here as those whose age at onset was under 21) are a distinct minority of those who are deaf or have serious trouble hearing.

Sex, Illness, and Limitation of Activity

The most recent demographic profile, drawn from the 1977 NHIS, shows that hearing trouble is proportionately overrepresented among males, whites, persons in families earning under $7,000 a year, and those with less than 12 years of education (Table 1-10). Among different age groups, most of these relationships are in the same direction but of lesser magnitude. This is especially true for family income and education, because lesser income and education are associated with advancing age that is highly associated with poorer hearing. People with trouble hearing were also overrepresented in the South and outside standard metropolitan statistical areas.

Because of the close association of advancing age with both hearing loss and ill health, it is not surprising that people with a hearing loss are far less healthy than those with normal hearing. Yet the relationship between hearing loss and poor health holds when age is held constant. In all age groups, persons with a hearing loss were more likely than those with good hearing to contact a doctor more than five times a year, to spend over seven days a year in bed due to illness or disability, and to have their activity limited by a chronic condition (Table 1-11).

A "limitation of activity due to chronic conditions" is the NHIS concept that most closely resembles the more widely used term "disabled." Only 12 per cent of persons over 2 years old with normal hearing, compared with 61 per cent of those with serious trouble hearing, were limited in activity; the difference remains substantial in each age group examined (Table 1-11).

None of the health-related characteristics shown in Table 1-11 and discussed to this point refer specifically to the effects of hearing loss.

Text continued on page 20

Table 1-8. Number of Persons 25-74 Years, by Better-Ear Average Hearing Level for 500, 1000, and 2000 Hertz, Mean Hearing Level, and Standard Error, by Age: United States, 1974-1975

Age	Better-Ear Average in Decibels* of Persons 25-74 Years Old (in Thousands)									Standard Error of Mean
	All Levels	Less than 26	26 to 40	41 to 55	56 to 70	71 to 90	91 or more	Unknown	Mean†	
All	108,494	99,023	6,204	1,330	685	387	111	753	11.1	0.41
25-34	29,682	29,105	197	39	—	66	—	274	5.4	0.28
35-44	22,360	21,725	337	134	21	26	—	117	7.9	0.27
45-54	23,550	21,898	1,063	166	86	82	55	200	11.2	0.50
55-64	19,479	16,840	1,941	460	124	14	44	55	15.7	0.74
65-74	13,423	9,454	2,667	531	454	199	12	107	21.9	1.12

— Data not available.

* Re audiometric zero, American National Standards Institute, 1969; excludes those with one or more missing hearing levels at 500, 1000, or 2000 Hz.

†All persons with hearing levels of 100 dB or more were coded "99"; the distribution of average hearing levels for the better ear will reflect this truncation.

Source: Preliminary data from National Health and Nutrition Examination Survey.

Table 1-9. Number of Persons 3 Years of Age and Older with Bilateral Hearing Loss, by Age at Onset, Speech Comprehension Group, and Age; Percentage with Bilateral Hearing Loss with Onset under 21 Years, by Speech Comprehension Group and Age: United States, 1971

Ages 3 Years and Older	All Ages of Onset			Onset Under 21 Years of Age			Onset Under 21 Years of Age as a Percentage of All Ages at Onset		
	All Speech Comprehension Groups*	At Best Can Hear Shouted Speech	Can Hear Normal Speech	All Speech Comprehension Groups*	At Best Can Hear Shouted Speech	Can Hear Normal Speech	All Speech Comprehension Groups*	At Best Can Hear Shouted Speech	Can Hear Normal Speech
	Number of Persons in Thousands						Per Cent		
	6,414	2,447	3,878	1,386	588	784	21.6	24.0	20.2
3-16	394	151	240	394	151	240	100.0	100.0	100.0
17-44	829	217	599	457	143	308	55.1	65.9	51.4
45-64	1,845	556	1,262	294	138	151	15.9	24.8	12.0
65 and over	3,347	1,523	1,777	241	155	85	7.2	10.2	4.8

* Includes unknown hearing scale scores.

From Gentile, A. (1971). *Persons with impaired hearing, United States, 1971*. National Center for Health Statistics. Washington, DC: U.S. Government Printing Office.

Table 1-10. Per Cent Distribution of Persons 3 Years of Age and Older by Sociodemographic Characteristics, Age, and Hearing Ability: United States, 1977

Age and Hearing Ability	Total*	Sex		Race		Family Income			Years of Education Completed		
		Male	Female	White	Black	Under $7,000	$7,000–$14,999	$15,000 and over	Less than 12	12	More than 12
					Per Cent Distribution						
All 3 years and over											
No trouble hearing	100	48	53	88	12	21	33	47	30	38	32
All levels of hearing trouble	100	57	43	93	7	37	31	32	50	28	22
At best can hear shouted speech	100	56	44	94	6	47	29	24	66	21	13
3–44											
No trouble hearing	100	49	51	87	13	18	34	49	20	41	39
All levels of hearing trouble	100	62	38	91	9	20	37	43	24	39	37
At best can hear shouted speech	100	58	42	88	12	26	37	37	28	44	27
45–64											
No trouble hearing	100	46	54	90	10	18	30	52	37	39	24
All levels of hearing trouble	100	63	37	94	6	25	32	44	45	34	22
At best can hear shouted speech	100	68	32	96	4	29	36	36	54	31	15
Over 64											
No trouble hearing	100	38	62	90	10	53	30	17	60	22	18
All levels of hearing trouble	100	49	51	94	6	60	26	14	68	18	14
At best can hear shouted speech	100	50	50	95	5	61	24	15	76	14	10

* Excludes persons other than white or black and unknown family income and education.

From Ries, P. W. (1982). *Hearing ability of persons by sociodemographic and health characteristics: United States* (Series 10, No. 140). National Center for Health Statistics. Washington, DC: U.S. Government Printing Office.

Table 1-11.   Per Cent Distribution of Persons 3 Years of Age and Older by Selected Health Characteristics, Age, and Hearing Ability: United States, 1977

Age and Hearing Ability	Annual Physician Contacts*			Annual Bed Disability Days†			Limitation of Activity and Hearing Trouble as a Cause of Limitation				
									Hearing Trouble		
	None	1-5 Contacts	5 or More Contacts	None	1-7 Days	8 or More Days	Not Limited	Limited	Main Cause	Secondary Cause	Not Listed as Cause
	Per Cent Distribution										
All over 2 years											
No trouble hearing	26	58	16	55	34	11	88	12	—	—	—
All levels of hearing trouble	17	53	30	51	27	21	58	42	7	5	88
At best can hear shouted speech	16	49	36	51	22	28	39	61	12	8	80
3–44											
No trouble hearing	26	60	14	52	39	9	94	6	—	—	—
All levels of hearing trouble	19	56	24	41	42	17	78	22	27	5	68
At best can hear shouted speech	15	56	29	39	39	22	50	50	49	5‡	45
45–64											
No trouble hearing	26	54	20	61	25	14	79	21	—	—	—
All levels of hearing trouble	18	53	29	52	27	21	60	40	6	4	91
At best can hear shouted speech	17	47	36	53	21	26	46	54	14	7‡	79
Over 64											
No trouble hearing	21	51	28	65	17	18	62	38	—	—	—
All levels of hearing trouble	15	51	34	58	18	24	44	56	3	5	92
At best can hear shouted speech	15	48	37	52	18	30	34	66	6	8	86

* Excludes unknown annual physician contacts.
† Excludes unknown annual days in bed.
‡ Estimate has a relative standard error of over 30 per cent.
From Ries, P. W. (1982). *Hearing ability of persons by sociodemographic and health characteristics: United States.* (Series 10, No. 140). National Center for Health Statistics. Washington, DC: U.S. Government Printing Office.

Respondents whom NHIS classified as limited in activity were asked to list up to three conditions which caused the limitation and, if more than one was listed, to specify which was the main cause. Relatively few persons—12 per cent of those with any hearing trouble and 20 per cent of those with a serious hearing loss—cited it as a cause of their limitation.

These findings were strongly affected by age. Among persons with a serious hearing loss, only 6 per cent of those over 64 years of age but 49 per cent of those 3 to 44 years old cited their loss as the main cause of their limitations. This relationship resembles that shown in Table 1-9 between present age, age at onset, and the degree of hearing loss. The hearing loss of many younger persons is their major health-related problem, whereas that of many older persons is only one of several health-related problems.

The picture that emerges from this brief profile of hearing-impaired persons is in many ways similar to that of an underprivileged minority. Both groups are proportionately overrepresented among those in poor health and lower socioeconomic groups. However, because of high mortality and birth rates, underprivileged groups are generally young, whereas the hearing-impaired are comparatively old. The problems of the aged and hearing-impaired populations appear to be linked in important ways. The growing proportion of older persons in the national population implies a growing prevalence of hearing impairment and, presumably, a growing need for appropriate medical, audiological, and rehabilitation services to alleviate these impairments.

REFERENCES

Feller, B. (1981). *Prevalence of selected impairments, United States, 1977* (Series 10, No. 134). National Center for Health Statistics. Washington, DC: U.S. Government Printing Office.

Gentile, A. (1971). *Persons with impaired hearing, United States, 1971* (Series 10, No. 101). National Center for Health Statistics. Washington, DC: U.S. Government Printing Office.

Glorig, A., and Roberts, J. (1965). *Hearing levels of adults by age and sex, United States, 1960-1962* (Series 11, No. 11). National Center for Health Statistics. Washington, DC: U.S. Government Printing Office.

Ries, P. W. (1982). *Hearing ability of persons by sociodemographic and health characteristics: United States* (Series 10, No. 140). National Center for Health Statistics. Washington, DC: U.S. Government Printing Office.

Roberts, J., and Ahuja, E. M. (1975). *Hearing levels of youths 12-17 years, United States* (Series 11, No. 145). National Center for Health Statistics. Washington, DC: U.S. Government Printing Office.

Roberts, J., and Haber, P. (1970). *Hearing levels of children by age and sex, United States* (Series 11, No. 102). National Center for Health Statistics. Washington, DC: U.S. Government Printing Office.

Schein, J. (n.d.). *Revision of the Gallaudet hearing scale: Clinical phase.* Mimeographed, Gallaudet College, Washington, DC.

Schein, J., and Delk, M., Jr. (1974). *The deaf population of the United States.* Silver Spring, MD: National Association of the Deaf.

Schein, J., Gentile, A., and Haase, K. W. (1970). *Development and evaluation of an expanded hearing loss scale questionnaire* (Series 2, No. 37). National Center for Health Statistics. Washington, DC: U.S. Government Printing Office.

Wilder, C. (1975). *Prevalence of selected impairments, United States, 1971* (Series 10, No. 99). National Center for Health Statistics. Washington, DC: U.S. Government Printing Office.

Chapter **2**
Older Adults: Social and Economic Conditions

George L. Maddox, Jr.

As noted in Chapter 1, a large proportion of adults with hearing problems are elderly. While they are learning to adjust to hearing losses they must also deal with numerous other aspects of aging, which may influence the adjustment process.

Aging as a personal concern is ancient. Aging as a societal concern is relatively recent and as a scientific concern is more recent still. Nevertheless, four decades of social commentary and scientific research have generated a large and expanding literature that, at best, can be highlighted only selectively. Specifying the three specific objectives of this chapter is, therefore, particularly important.

First, attention will be given to three interrelated revolutions in our understanding of personal and societal aging—the demographic revolution, the knowledge revolution, and the revolution in conceptualizing the future of aging and future research about aging. Both society and the scientific community have been rethinking their understanding of human aging.

Second, a succinct review of social science research evidence about the current and future social and economic status of older adults in the United States will be provided. In this context a few comparative observations about aging in other societies will be introduced for purposes of illustration. However, the focus here is primarily on the United States.

Third, the chapter will conclude with some limited observations about hearing loss in later life. These observations will be limited by a relative scarcity of information, not about the incidence and prevalence of hearing loss in the later years, but about the consequences and implications of this loss.

THREE INTERRELATED REVOLUTIONS IN THINKING ABOUT AGING

The Demographic Revolution

While counting and projecting the number of older adults in our society is important, these activities have tended to become somewhat ritualistic, banal, unproductive, and diverting exercises. Certain important points tend to be missed when journalists and scientists view with alarm evidence of population aging. Three critical but often neglected issues are raised by the demographics of aging populations.

1. Epidemiological information about the relationship between age and disease, impairment, and disability or handicap—not just numbers of older persons—is the basis of real concern. Large numbers of functionally competent individuals do not have the same implications for society as large numbers of functionally impaired, dependent persons. The factual basis for assessing the relationship between age and functional impairment is far more ambiguous than it need or should be. This ambiguity is at the heart of what I have called the Fries-anti-Fries debate (Fries, 1980; Schneider and Brody, 1983) regarding whether, as Fries contends, the onset of functional impairment is being—or can be—delayed as average life expectancy increases. The absence of definitive evidence is fueling a passionate but inconclusive debate about whether the future of an aging society is worse or better than we expect.

2. Current institutional arrangements for meeting essential welfare and health needs of an aging population are mismatched with the demands of older adults. Social security, widely regarded as one of the great pieces of legislation in American history, was not designed to insure an adequate level of income for an aging population expected to live two decades past retirement, inclined to retire before age 65, and with the experience of high rates of both unemployment and inflation. Health care, which focuses primarily on medical care in hospitals, is mismatched with the needs of older adults for a substantial amount of primary, preventive, rehabilitative, and community-based care. The housing that serves middle-aged adults is mismatched with the needs of older adults. Access to essential services remains largely dependent on private transportation. And education continues to be designed primarily for the young.

3. The provision of care for seriously impaired older adults remains the responsibility mainly of the private sector (particularly of family members), which bears 80 per cent of the cost, whereas the public sector provides only 20 per cent (Laurie, 1978). Personal responsibility for the provision of care falls heavily on middle-aged women who, to an increasing degree, are entering the labor force. The implications of these facts are

poorly understood and have been inadequately considered in the formation of public policy.

The Knowledge Revolution

In the past four decades, significant advances in scientific knowledge
about the biological, behavioral, and social processes of aging have occurred. Scientific advances are not only appearing in gerontological journals but, increasingly, in the major journals of all relevant disciplines. We
are now beyond the stage of describing aging process and at the point of
implementing one of the most basic maxims of the experimental and
clinical sciences: *If you want to understand a process, try to change it.*

For example, through biomedical research, understanding the bio-
chemistry of cellular functioning has led to new and more precise understanding of how both nutrition and therapeutic drugs modify the risk of
disease and functioning in later life. We now understand the potential
health benefits of aerobic exercise even for very old adults.

Through behavioral research, we now know that significant loss of
memory and cognitive functioning is not a normal concomitant of aging in
the absence of disease. Older adults can be taught adaptive skills that
increase the probability of independent functioning.

Through social science research, we know that environmental stimu-
lation and opportunities for social interaction are important determinants
of adult behavior. Environments that demand too much or too little are
detrimental for older adults. Matching levels of functional capacity and
environmental demand becomes particularly important in later life.

For summary discussions of these conclusions see Maddox and Wiley
(1976), Maddox and Campbell (1984), and Maddox (1985). The last
paper reviews a virtual revolution in current scientific thinking about the
mutability of aging processes and hence the potential of guided intervention to construct the future of aging differently. Attention is also called to
the recent work of Arnetz (1983) in Sweden, which documents the
consequences of understimulation in later life. This work is of particular
relevance in understanding the possible implications of hearing loss, a
prevalent cause of sensory understimulation in later life.

The Revolution of Realistic Expectation and Hope

Each successive cohort of adults is arriving at age 65 better educated,
in better health, and with more secure retirement incomes. In the United
States, older persons have been more active politically than other adults;
increasingly, they and those who speak for them appear to understand how

the political process works and are using this understanding to become a force in American politics.

The Federal government has been responsive, for example, with the Older Americans Act, Medicare, the creation of the National Institute on Aging, and legislation designed to enhance employment at least until age 70.

Professional societies have been responsive by ensuring that both basic and continuing education includes exposure to gerontology and geriatrics. Proportionately, the United States has more individuals trained in gerontology and geriatrics than any other nation.

All this does not lead to the conclusion that enough is being done to safeguard the future of an aging society. Clearly, however, both lay persons and professionals now tend to share a common view of aging. Aging processes are perceived as modifiable, not immutable. The future of aging can be constructed differently and, hopefully, in beneficial ways.

SOCIAL PROFILE OF OLDER ADULTS

This brief profile must necessarily be sketched with broad strokes. Detailed documentation can be found in Maddox and Campbell (1985) and Maddox and Wiley (1976). Underlying the profile is also 20 years of research in the Duke Longitudinal Studies of Aging (1982).

Variation

The earlier literature on aging—commonly and even current literature occasionally—refers to older adults as *the elderly*. Such a designation is at odds with the evidence and invites misunderstanding. Variance in the characteristics of older adults is considerable; older adults do not become more alike as they age. In the long run they are all dead, but their routes to that end differ considerably.

Consider, for example, age. Adults between ages 65 and 90 comprise five five-year cohorts, each with a distinctly different profile of educational attainment, functional capacity, sex ratio, and economic security. Older adults of the same age are equidistant from birth but not from death. Older women, on the average, outlive older men. Older adults of higher and lower socioeconomic status experience later life differently.

The known differences among older adults have led some students of aging to distinguish the "young old" and "old old" and to stress the importance of a differential gerontology. In the United Kingdom, geriatric patients are defined as 75 years of age or older out of recognition that they have a distinctly higher probability of significant functional impairment than do younger persons.

Or, consider economic resources. Conventional wisdom associates old age with a high risk of poverty. Current economic research presents a far more complex and benign picture. The incidence of poverty in later life is now about the same as among all adults. Taking income transfers into account, about 6 per cent of older adults are poor. The determination of poverty is controversial and, however defined, poverty is not to be excused. But not all older people are impoverished; the majority have adequate incomes; some are rich. Poverty is more likely to be experienced by those in minority groups and very old women (Clark, Maddox, Schrimper, and Sumner, 1984).

Consider functional capacity and impairment. The great majority of older persons live out their lives in the community competently and with personal satisfaction. They are not characteristically isolated, sick, and depressed. At any one time, about 5 per cent are institutionalized (typically in long-term care facilities); over a lifetime, about 20 per cent are. At any one time, at least twice as many (10 per cent) older adults living at home are as functionally impaired as those in institutions.

Information from the Duke Older Americans Resources and Services (OARS) research (Maddox and Dellinger, 1978) in various sites across the nation provides additional insight into the multiple dimensions of impairment. For example, OARS estimates that about 15 to 20 per cent of persons over age 64 living in the community are impaired in their capacity for self-care; 12 to 14 per cent are impaired mentally, and 25 to 28 per cent are impaired physically. About 9 to 11 per cent lack essential social support to ensure informal care.

If the most vulnerable older adults are defined as those with a significant impairment in capacity for self-care or in physical *or* mental functioning *and* without having either economic or social resources to compensate, the OARS evidence suggests that about 2 per cent of older adults in the community are in this "most vulnerable" category. The risk of all impairments increases with age and is higher for persons with low incomes.

Continuities in the Life Course

The past is, indeed, prologue. The experience of old age reflects previous experience that has created different social and economic resources, different lifestyles that affect health, and different adaptive skills that affect responses to challenging life events.

Not surprisingly, economically secure older adults tend to live longer than their poor counterparts and are more likely to report a higher level of perceived well-being and satisfaction with retirement and to have adequate social supports when support is needed. Well-educated older persons are more likely than those with little education to adapt successfully to stressful life events.

To arrive at age 65 with a history of a "risky lifestyle" characterized by poor nutrition, cigarette smoking, poor skills for adapting to stress, inactivity, ignorance, poverty, and social isolation has fatal implications for survival and the maintenance of well-being.

Mobilization of Potential

The bad news of arriving at age 65 with limited personal and social resources is offset by some good news. As already noted, each successive cohort of adults reaching age 65 appears to have more personal and social resources. Age-specific life expectancy continues to increase. Scientific knowledge about how to compensate for age-related impairments is improving. Interest in personal reduction of risks through changes in lifestyle is increasing.

While science is a long way from being able to promise immortality or even an impairment-free old age, new evidence is accumulating to suggest greater potential for modifying functional capacity in the later years than was suspected even a decade ago. Preventive health measures in the adult years, geriatric medicine, and appropriate matching of individual capacity and situational opportunity are contributing to a new, realistic sense of our capacity to modify aging processes and construct the later years differently.

As noted previously, this optimistic view is not universally shared. Participants in the Fries-anti-Fries debate are in disagreement about the evidence regarding the reduction of morbidity as life expectancy increases.

Environments

Differential aging and differences in the experience of aging are partly determined by genetics. Clearly, however, more than genetics is required to explain observed differences. Social science research has documented variances in aging processes and the experience of aging that cannot possibly be explained by genetic variation alone.

Societies have different material resources and allocate them differently. Populations in poor societies in the developing world have life expectancies considerably below those in the richer developed world. The probability of survival into later life is, in part, a function of economic resources; average life expectancy rises as resources increase. The pessimistic view that modernization inevitably leads to loss of status and reduced well-being in older adults has been contradicted by evidence from comparative studies.

Within a particular society, survival and well-being are a function of the distribution of resources. Placement within the stratification system as indexed by education, occupation, and income affects survival and well-being in the adult and later years. In the United States, research has demonstrated that unhealthy, risky lifestyles and behavior are more common among lower than higher status individuals. Certain correlates of lower status, such as social isolation, ignorance, poverty, and poor nutrition, are themselves conditions that increase the risk of impairment, ineffective coping behavior, disease, and death.

When we seek to improve the health and well-being of older adults, we think of improving their health care. It is more difficult for us to understand the potential contribution of improved income, housing, transportation, and education to the well-being of older adults (Maddox, 1985).

The immediate environments, or milieus, of older adults are also important in understanding their behavior. Of particular importance are the special living environments of impaired older adults. Social allocation processes have a rather high probability of mismatching individuals with varying levels of competence with appropriate milieus that encourage a maximum feasible amount of personal independence. Improving the match of individual and milieu is possible and, when it occurs, beneficial outcomes follow. We know theoretically how to achieve improved matching, but we have not mastered the practical politics of doing so.

HEARING LOSS

Ries (1982), at the National Center for Health Statistics (NCHS), published the most definitive statement currently available on the epidemiology of hearing ability and its sociodemographic correlates in the United States. Reporting findings from the use of the Gallaudet Hearing Scale in a number of large surveys, Ries concluded that hearing loss competes with loss of teeth as the nation's most prevalent impairment. This generalization also applies to Sweden (Arnetz, 1983); limitation of hearing is almost eight times more common, for example, than limitation of vision (26.5 per 100 versus 3.6 per 100) among persons 65 years of age and older in that country.

Ries documents that hearing impairment increases with age in the United States. For persons over 64 years of age, the prevalence of some hearing trouble in 1977 was 26.9 per 100 (31.4 for men; 22.6 for women), and the prevalence of severe hearing loss (Gallaudet Scale scores 3 to 8), 16.5 per 100 (20.6 for men; 13.5 for women). Swedish estimates are comparable (Arnetz, 1983).

In its Health Insurance Experiment studies, Rand Corporation (1981) focused on the conceptualization and measurement of hearing loss in adults up to age 64. Using a better ear threshold of 26 dB as "within the normal range," the study found that measured hearing loss and severity of loss both increased with age. The estimated hearing impairment "outside the normal range" of 10.6 per 100 for those 55 to 64 years old was three times higher than for those 35 to 44 years of age. If this change is extrapolated by a factor reflecting observed increasing hearing loss with age, the resulting estimate of hearing loss would appear to be in the range of 26.9 per 100 estimated from self-reports of individuals over age 64 that were summarized by Ries.

Wax (1983) concludes from a review of evidence that "a majority of people over 65 suffer the biological disruption of hearing loss serious enough to contribute to communication and other psychosocial difficulties among this age group." This estimate of prevalence of significant hearing loss is essentially double the estimate of self-reported and measured evidence presented above. Intuitively, however, Wax's conclusion is believable since the experience and significance of hearing loss surely reflect a subjective interpretation of how much loss is personally and socially tolerable. It should also be noted that Wax stresses "biological disruption of hearing loss," which is a warning that apparent hearing loss can and does reflect motivated "not hearing" as well as demonstrable biological loss. This distinction has not, so far as I know, been carefully studied.

The sociodemographic correlates of hearing loss reported by Ries follow a familiar pattern. Hearing loss is associated with lower education, lower income, and poorer health.

The Ries report does not estimate whether observed hearing loss is correctable with a hearing aid. The use of hearing aids was, however, reported. Among persons over age 64, 20 per cent of those with all levels of hearing loss and 37 per cent of those with severe losses reported using a hearing aid. Although the proportion with a correctable loss is not clear, it seems that a higher proportion could have their hearing improved by medical or surgical means or mechanical compensation.

The Ries study does not document the personal and social consequences of hearing loss for older adults beyond noting the association between loss and an elevated utilization of health care services and difficulty in conducting usual activities. It is easy to imagine how hearing loss disrupts interpersonal communication and restricts normal activities. Further, given the known deleterious consequences of understimulation of older adults, loss of hearing constitutes an obvious example of chronic understimulation (Arnetz, 1983). The Duke Longitudinal Studies of Aging documented correlates of pathology in the organization of personality related to hearing loss that was found to have negative consequences, more negative in fact than loss of sight (Eisdorfer, 1960a, 1960b; Eisdorfer and Wilkie, 1974). The negative impact was manifest in projective tests as increased rigidity, restricted interpretation of information, and primitive thought.

The Wax article (1983) is a pertinent illustration of one of the major arguments of this paper and provides an appropriate final comment: If one wants to understand an age-associated loss in function, try to change it. The particular intervention Wax discusses—involving impaired older persons in reading and writing poetry to enhance the personal meaning of life cycle change—expresses the new realistic basis for believing that one does not have to accept the implications of observed loss as though they are unmodifiable. There are now sufficient reasons to assert that correction or compensation for most hearing loss is possible. The decision to try to modify observed hearing loss is based in part on scientific evidence; but the decision to try to construct the experience of aging differently by actually attempting to reduce hearing loss goes beyond science to focus on personal and social values and intentions.

REFERENCES

Arnetz, B. (1983). *Psychosocial effects of understimulation in old age.* Stockholm: Karolinska Institute.

Clark, R., Maddox, G., Schrimper, R., and Sumner, D. (1984). *Inflation and the economic well-being of the elderly.* Baltimore: Johns Hopkins University Press.

Duke Longitudinal Studies of Aging Staff. An Overview of Outcomes (1982). The Duke Multidisciplinary Longitudinal Studies of Normal Aging (whole issue). *Duke University Center Advances in Research, 6.*

Eisdorfer, C. (1960a). Developmental level sensory impairment in the aged. *Journal of Projective Techniques and Personality Assessment, 24,* 129-132.

Eisdorfer, C. (1960b). Rorschach rigidity and sensory decrement in a senescent population. *Journal of Gerontology, 15,* 188-190.

Eisdorfer, C., and Wilkie, F. (1974). Auditory change. In E. Palmore (Ed.), *Normal aging, II* (pp. 32-41). Durham, NC: Duke University Press.

Fries, J. (1980). Aging, natural death, and the compression of morbidity. *New England Journal of Medicine, 303,* 130-135.

Laurie, W. (1978). Employing the Duke OARS methodology in cost comparisons: Home services and institutionalization (whole issue). *Duke University Center Advances in Research, 2.*

Maddox, G. (1985). Intervention strategies to enhance well-being in later life: The status and prospects of guided change. *Health Services Research, 19* (Supplement), 6.

Maddox, G., and Campbell, R. (1985). Scope, concepts, and methods in the study of aging. In R. Binstock and E. Shanas (Eds.), *The handbook of aging and the social sciences* (2nd edition). New York: Van Nostrand Reinhold.

Maddox, G., and Dellinger, D. (1978). Assessment of functional status in a program evaluation and resource allocation model. *Annals of the American Academy of Political and Social Science, 438,* 59-70.

Maddox, G., and Wiley, J. (1976). Scope, concepts and methods in the study of aging. In R. Binstock and E. Shanas (Eds.), *The handbook of aging and the social sciences.* New York: Van Nostrand Reinhold.

Rand Corporation (1981). *Conceptualization and measurement of physiologic health of adults: Hearing loss* (Vol. 14). Santa Monica, CA: Author.

Ries, P. W. (1982). *Hearing ability of persons by sociodemographic and health characteristics: United States* (Series 10, No. 140). National Center for Health Statistics. Washington, DC: U.S. Government Printing Office.

Schneider, E., and Brody, J. (1983). Aging, natural death, and the compression of morbidity: Another view. *New England Journal of Medicine, 309,* 854-855.

Wax, T. (1983). Poetry efforts by aged deaf: Expression of life cycle experience. *Gerontologist, 23,* 462-466.

PART II

SOCIAL AND PSYCHOLOGICAL EFFECTS OF HEARING LOSS

Chapter **3**

Social and Psychological Effects of Hearing Loss in Adulthood: A Literature Review

Kathryn P. Meadow-Orlans

> We deafened people have two lives: the years with ears and the years without. We pass from one to the other over a bridge of sighs or on stepping-stones of self-determination. It all depends. (Heiner, p. 13)

Those factors determining the "sighs" and the "self-determination"—the individual's responses to deafness in the adult years—are the subject of this chapter. Depending on a social scientist's theoretical orientation or a layman's personal philosophy, explanations of these responses may emphasize human nature, character, early childhood experiences, income, family and community support, societal attitudes, or role relationships. Without doubt, the nature of the hearing loss and the availability of technical aids also affect reactions to that loss.

I will first review the characteristics of adult hearing loss which most affect the individual's responses. Next, I will consider the psychological consequences of hearing loss and the personality traits that affect them. Finally, I will discuss some social consequences and social factors. A separate section deals with hearing loss in elderly persons. I have attempted to combine a review of the research literature with illustrations and insights drawn from personal documents.

NATURE OF THE HEARING LOSS

It is surprising how often scholars have confused those individuals who became deaf before they acquired speech, and who may or may not use sign language, with the much larger population of deafened adults, whose experience and problems differ radically. Even prominent social scientists such as Roger Barker (1953) and Karl Menninger failed to make this crucial distinction. As Thomas (1981, p. 219) observed, "Even researchers have sometimes failed to grasp the distinction" in selecting subjects. This chapter will be confined to a discussion of the post-vocationally deafened, defined here as those whose hearing is impaired at age 25 or later. Within this population, it is necessary to consider the age at onset, the degree of impairment, the rapidity of onset, and the shape of the hearing loss or residual hearing.

Age at Onset

To evaluate the impact of deafness we should know the individual's current age and age at onset. The meaning of hearing loss at various points in the life cycle is summarized by one research group who investigated onset in elderly persons:

> Attitudes to a disorder first suffered at a stage in life when it was felt to be untimely and exceptional are different from the response to the same disorder encountered at a stage where it is conventionally expected as part of a "normal running down" and indeed has become . . . a norm. (Humphrey, Gilhome-Herbst, and Faurqi, 1981, p. 29)

Severity of Loss

It seems obvious that the effects of hearing loss are related to its severity. Nonetheless, many studies have disregarded this point and have included subjects whose hearing was within the normal range. Just how the loss is measured—by pure tone averages, speech threshold tests, word lists, self-reports, interviewer assessments, or audiometric tests with and without hearing aids—is a separate, albeit important, question. Clearly, the degree of functional hearing loss has a great effect on an individual's ability to adjust to the loss. *

---

* There is a considerable volume of literature on hearing scales designed to assess the extent of hearing loss and how it affects communication and social interaction from answers to a series of questions. Efforts have been made to validate some scales by audiological tests; the value and comparability of different studies will obviously rest upon the validity and reliability of the scales employed. Unfortunately, the scales have not been adequately and comprehensively evaluated, although Rosen (1979) makes an effort to do so.

Among the scales most frequently used are the Gallaudet Hearing Scale (Schein, 1968, pp. 8-14; Schein, Gentile, and Haase, 1970; Schein and Delk, 1974, pp. 134-138), the Social Hearing Handicap Index (Ewertsen and Birk-Nielsen, 1973), and the Hearing Measure scale (Noble and Atherly, 1970). More recently, the Hearing Handicap Inventory for the Elderly has been published (Ventry and Weinstein, 1982).

Giolas (1982, pp. 50-77) provides a helpful discussion of these scales and reprints four that are not readily available: the Hearing Handicap Scale (High, Fairbanks, and Glorig, 1964), the Denver Scale of Communication Function (Alpiner et al., 1974), the Hearing Performance Inventory (Giolas, Owens, Lamb, and Schubert, 1979), and the Denver Scale of Communication Function for Senior Citizens Living in Retirement Centers (Zarnoch and Alpiner, 1976).

Rapidity of Loss

Reactions to hearing loss are also influenced by its gradualness or rapidity. Mulrooney (1973, p. 37), deafened suddenly in an automobile accident, stresses "grief as a response to loss" in describing her experience. Elliott (1978), a deafened woman, makes a related point in recounting a conversation with a prelingually deaf man, who said, "I'm better off than you are. You lost something, I didn't." She replied, "Maybe I'm better off. I had something, you didn't." Another deafened person writes that becoming deaf

> ... can take considerable time and prove a long, drawn out incredibly cruel and anxiety-filled process. And it can, as in my case, happen very quickly and be all over within a few days. But no matter how it happens, it is a major watershed in one's life. To become deaf as an adult is to be cut off in the midst of one's dreams and plans for the future, whatever they may be. Life comes to a halt. (Anderson, 1981, p. 70)

Residual Hearing

Depending on the level of frequencies of residual hearing, it may be more or less possible to provide a hearing aid for sounds in the speech range or, failing that, for grosser environmental sounds. Tinnitus—unremitting or recurrent ringing or rasping ear noises—often distracts and distresses deafened adults. The phenomenon of recruitment, which makes certain sounds unbearably loud, can also make it difficult for hearing persons to understand the deafened person's reactions. Thus, the audiological, social, and psychological dimensions of hearing loss are intertwined.

Brooks (1979) summarizes five English studies reported over a ten year period: all suggest that only a minority of those with impaired hearing use hearing aids. Her own research indicated that this pattern was difficult to change. "It was depressing to find that even after counseling the amount of use made of the hearing aids by [our] patients was only about one or two hours per day . . . mainly for watching TV." Usage was unrelated to sex and living arrangements but appeared greater with severe impairment (p. 107).

Summary

The population of those with a hearing loss after age 24 is composed of important subgroups based upon the age of onset, its sudden or progressive character, its severity, and the nature of any residual hearing.

PSYCHOLOGICAL EFFECTS

Several primary symptoms, diagnoses, or descriptions of deafened persons are discussed in the clinical and research literature.* In some respects, conclusions are contradictory. Frequently there are problems of representativeness, attentiveness to the subgroups noted above, and appropriate measurements. The literature deals with (1) paranoia; (2) depression, withdrawal, and isolation; and (3) irritability, fatigue, and nervousness.

Paranoia

Despite a persistent myth that deafened persons are likely to develop symptoms of paranoia, the research evidence is contradictory.

Interviews and tests of 378 patients at the audiology clinic of the University of Pittsburgh Medical School were reported by Nett (1960). The patients had a mean hearing level of 33 decibels (the mean of 42 per cent was under 30 dB) and 70 per cent had never used a hearing aid. In the Minnesota Multiphasic Personality Inventory (MMPI), 78 per cent were within the normal range for "hysteria"; 82 per cent, within the normal range for "depression"; 90 and 83 per cent, respectively, within the normal range for "paranoia" and "hypochondria" (p. 44). Depending on which of six measures of hearing loss was utilized, the correlation (*eta* coefficient) between the "paranoia" scale score and hearing loss ranged from .22 ("six ordered frequencies") to a high of .79 ("AMA [American Medical Association] percentage loss") (p. 99).

Commenting on the Nett study, Thomas (1981) suggests that use of the *eta* coefficient might have led to spurious conclusions. Perhaps a more telling criticism is the uncritical use of the MMPI, with items prejudicial to a deafened person, such as "I am easily awakened by noise," "I would like to be a singer," "My speech is the same as always," "I find it hard to make talk when I meet new people," and "My hearing is apparently as good as most people."

Myklebust (1964) studied individuals deafened in adulthood who were members of speechreading classes at a hearing society. The 44 men, mean age 39, had a mean hearing loss of 68 dB; the 83 women, mean age 50, a mean loss of 66 dB. Analyzing the MMPI responses with and without items

---

*I have omitted some of the more technical psychoanalytic studies in this chapter; thus I have not considered responses such as compensation, denial, projection, or the "sexual significance" of hearing and deafness. Readers interested in these formulations may consult Rousey (1971) and Knapp (1960b).

"loaded" against deafened persons, he found the deafened men more emotionally maladjusted than hearing men on all scales *except* "paranoia." Their scores were most deviate, first, for schizophrenia and, second, for depression. The deafened women showed less maladjustment than the men (pp. 142-143).

Thomas and Gilhome-Herbst (1980) contacted all persons who first received a hearing aid from 1970 to 1976 at three clinics in the Greater London area. They interviewed 236 persons (48 per cent of those contacted), of whom two thirds were 50 or older and had a 40 to 69 dB hearing loss (pp. 77-78). Of those tested on a screening inventory designed to assess anxiety and depression, 19 per cent were judged psychiatrically disturbed, compared with 5 per cent of the general population and 75 per cent of psychiatric hospitalized patients ($p < .001$).

The authors believe that these figures underestimate the degree of psychiatric disability actually evidenced in their study group. The deafened subjects scored "worse" than hearing controls on physical disabilities, having enough energy, consulting a doctor about a nervous problem, satisfaction with their health, and "worry." They were much more likely to have other health problems in addition to deafness. The only questions which did *not* discriminate the deafened and hearing subjects were three designed to measure suspiciousness (p. 78). The authors feel that this argues strongly against a high prevalence of paranoia in deafened persons.

Cooper and his colleagues (1974; Kay, Cooper, Garside, and Roth, 1976) compared 65 mental hospital patients with paranoid psychosis and 67 patients with primary affective disorders. Significantly more of the former registered a pure tone hearing loss (none had early profound deafness). Of the paranoid patients 25, compared with 12 of those with affective disorders, were judged "socially deaf," defined as "difficulty in hearing speech in any part of a church or theater but able to hear speech at close range without an aid" (1974, p. 851).

Comparisons of the prevalence of various diagnoses among hospitalized patients, especially those with serious hearing loss, are problematic unless allowance is made for the different length of hospitalization for different conditions. Trybus (1983) has shown that the mean length of hospitalization for deaf patients was over 12 months in contrast to under 6 months for hearing patients. Hence, with equal rates of hospitalization per 1,000 deaf and hearing adults, the apparent rate, as measured by the relative number in hospital at any time, will be twice as high for deaf adults. After hospitalization, Zarit (1980) suggested that patients with severe hearing loss are less likely to be included in treatment groups because their presence may be "disruptive" (p. 331).

Primary and secondary diagnoses may vary widely depending on many factors. "Suspiciousness" is not, of course, the same as the clinical condition of "paranoia," as Heiner's (1949) report of her response to progressive deafness may illustrate. "When I saw two of my friends with their heads together, talking, I grew tense with suspicion. They must be talking about me because they seemed to be taking care that I should not hear what was said" (p. 47). A therapist observed:

> Not hearing speech clearly, especially in a group situation, the deaf person may conclude that others are talking about him, or may distort those bits of speech that are partially perceived. Similarly voices and intruders may provide some social stimulation to the isolated older person. A patient seen by the author had complained of hearing voices, which had become threatening. Following treatment . . . she stated that she knew she had made up these voices, because she missed the sounds of human conversation. (Zarit, 1980, p. 219)

Summary

The evidence from the preceding studies is equivocal. Most conclude that deafened persons are more emotionally maladjusted than comparable hearing subjects. However, evidence for the specific diagnosis of paranoia is mixed indeed. Nett (1960) indicates that deafened persons are more likely to be paranoid, but her research is seriously flawed. Myklebust (1964) and Thomas and Gilhome-Herbst (1980) find the prevalence of paranoia no higher, whereas Cooper, Kay, Curry, Garside, and Roth (1974) find it higher in deafened individuals. It is easy to understand how a tendency to be "suspicious" of others' conversations could be labeled "paranoia" or expand to full-blown pathology.

Depression, Withdrawal, and Isolation

Many clinicians agree that depression and withdrawal with resultant isolation are the most prevalent psychological responses to severe hearing loss (but clinicians are not likely to see deafened people who do not become depressed). Research findings support these observations, as do reports from individuals who have experienced hearing loss. Beethoven's account is one of profound depression; Ellen Glasgow and others describe their sensitivity and fearfulness in society and eventual withdrawal from it:

> Oh you men who think that I am malevolent, stubborn, or misanthropic, how greatly do you wrong me. You do not know the secret cause which makes me seem that way to you. . . . If at times I tried to forget all this, oh how harshly was I flung back by the doubly sad experience of my bad hearing. Yet it was impossible for me to say to people, "Speak louder, shout, for I am deaf." . . . For me there can be no relaxation with my fellow men, no refined conversations, no mutual exchange of ideas. I must live almost alone, like one who has been banished . . . . I fear being exposed to the danger that my condition might be noticed . . . what a humiliation for me when someone standing next to me heard a flute in the distance and I heard nothing . . . . Such incidents drove me

almost to despair; a little more of that and I would have ended my life—it was only my art that held me back. (Beethoven, 1802, cited in Solomon, 1977, pp. 116-117)

For years now, ever since my deafness had begun to come nearer, I had felt as if I were waiting for an impenetrable wall to close round me. Meeting strangers had become torture, and I would go blocks out of my way to avoid a person I knew. (Glasgow, 1954, p. 181)

From 127 autobiographical accounts, Myklebust (1964) concluded that "social isolation was markedly apparent" in deafened adults, who were despondent and cynical about hearing persons (p. 131). He suggests that hearing loss can precipitate anxiety and depressive episodes in the elderly. "Usually the isolating effect of the inability to maintain contact auditorially can be readily recognized" (p. 121). Thomas and Gilhome-Herbst (1980) found loneliness more prevalent among deafened persons of employment age than among elderly persons; the moderately deaf felt as lonely as the severely deaf (p. 78).

Of 96 English subjects referred by physicians to hearing consultants, 20 per cent "dreaded" meeting new people, 14 per cent avoided meeting new people, and another 8 per cent would meet someone new only if accompanied by a hearing person (Beattie, 1981, p. 6). Interviews with 20 members of the Dutch Hard of Hearing Association were summarized as follows: "The image that tentatively emerges . . . is one of suffering, fear and loneliness" (Breed, van den Horst, and Mous, 1981, p. 316). With professional and personal experience of deafness in adulthood, Miller (1975) writes, "In the case of both the person who thinks of himself as hearing impaired and the one who does not, the greatest problem confronting him is his isolation . . . from social interaction . . . . [T]his type of isolation is a vicious circle, permitting the individual fewer and fewer opportunities for contact" (pp. 58-59).

Irritability, Fatigue, and Nervousness

Reports of nervousness, anxiety, heightened fearfulness, and irritability are common in accounts of deafened persons, professionals who work with them, and hearing persons with simulated deafness. Embarrassment is also frequently reported. These reactions may be more fleeting or situation-specific than paranoid or depressive symptoms.

Fatigue arises from trying to hear or lipread and to make oneself understood (Oyer and Oyer, 1979, p. 129). Fatigue, nervousness, and irritability are among the most noticeable effects of simulated deafness. In one experiment, two students with a 20 to 30 dB loss simulated with ear plugs were "tired, depressed and disliked making social contacts" (von der Lieth, 1972, p. 84). A group of students who wore plugs of ear mold material for 50 hours reported "unusual nervousness and tiredness." "I had to be on guard every minute in order to try to hear as much as possible." "I had to concentrate on watching their lips all the time" (Reichstein and von der Lieth, 1981, p. 303). A social worker notes that deafened persons seldom converse socially for more than an hour or two. "A deafened person is forever being surprised... caught unprepared. Nervousness, anxiety and fear are common experiences" (Luey, 1980, p. 258).

A deafened writer recalls: "Sometimes keeping up became so difficult for me that I, who used to laugh and chuckle all day long, became short-tempered and snappish—a crab!" (Heiner, 1949, p. 47). An audiologist describes clearly the interaction of several factors already noted:

> The individual feels disengaged from group interaction and apathy ensues, the product of the fatigue which sets in from the relentless effort of straining to hear. Frustration, kindled by begging too many pardons, gives way to subterfuges that disguise misunderstandings.... Finally, acquiescing to fatigue and frustration, thoughts stray from the conversation to mental imageries that are unburdened by the defective hearing mechanism. (Maurer, 1976, p. 60)

Empirical studies have less often noted such consequences of hearing loss. However, Thomas and Gilhome-Herbst (1980) found that deafened persons were significantly more likely than hearing controls to consult a doctor about nervous problems and worry (p. 80). When 500 new patients of a Department of Audiological Rehabilitation were asked to list the difficulties they had experienced, the largest proportion (48 per cent) cited hearing television and radio; 38 per cent cited general conversation; 14 per cent cited embarrassment; and 6 per cent cited nervousness (Stephens, 1980, pp. 208, 211).

SOCIAL EFFECTS

The social effects of later deafness will be discussed in four sections with much overlap among them: personal and group identity; work and career; family; and social aspects.

Personal and Group Identity

In personal accounts of acquired deafness, the sense of a changing self and the need to develop a new personal and social identity repeatedly emerge.

> Though the hard of hearing person may wear a hearing aid, he remains an auditory in between.... This [is] a question I have been asking myself all of my life. Where do I belong? ... in the world of the hearing or ... of the deaf? (McCartney, 1981, pp. 13-14)

A hard of hearing person who has faced his handicap and made an end to self-pity says to himself, "This is my country—this world of muffled sounds—often confusing, full of humiliating pitfalls. . . . I shall be living here all of my life . . . . These are my people." (Warfield, 1957, p. 64)

Even now I find myself wondering from time to time who I really am. Hearing people often think I am hearing because my speech is good; deaf people often think I am hearing because my signs are bad. Identity crisis. Hearing people have their culture based on spoken language and deaf people have their culture based on sign language and we are caught between incomprehensible speech on the one hand and incomprehensible signs on the other. If only those hearies would talk more clearly! If only those deafies would sign more slowly! (Elliott, 1978, p. 1)

A perceptive social worker entitles her paper on deafened adults "Between Worlds" (Luey, 1980). She believes it "almost inevitable" that the deafened person will lose some friends who will not submit to labored communication or who are "threatened or repelled by the sheer intensity of the deafened person's feelings" (p. 258). A survey of a discussion group of late-deafened adults found marginality and insecurity two of their most pressing problems: 86 per cent had made new friends; 50 per cent had been divorced; 68 per cent had changed career objectives, and 50 per cent had changed careers (Hunter, 1978).

Menninger (1952) discussed identity changes following disability in psychoanalytical terms of a body image that must be revised. He suggested that the deafened individual may experience a reawakening of "long-forgotten conflicts and associations with emotionally painful events and feelings of the past" (p. 11). Barker and Wright (1952) also discuss the changed body image that follows disablement, and they compare the disabled to an underprivileged racial or religious minority. "The non-disabled who value highly 'the body beautiful' may feel that in order for their value system to be maintained, those who suffer the loss of the body beautiful (or some other valued faculty) *must* feel devalued"—an attitude termed "the requirement of mourning" (p. 19). Nett (1960) argues that the minority group analogy, which "has so often in the past been used in connection with the cultural evaluation of handicap," is less pertinent than that of alienation in the special sense of self-estrangement:

Hearing handicapped persons in our society are treated not so much as a group different from, but as a class set apart from or forgotten by, the larger society. Thus their feelings are more of being alienated from others and of being excluded from activities they enjoy than of being discriminated against. (p. 117)

Thus, theorizing social scientists, clinicians, and deafened individuals agree that the redefinition of self is a dramatic necessity and that many hearing-impaired persons have a sense of "marginality" for years. An illuminating exception was observed in a study of 1,000 workers in two noisy factories in northern Sweden (Diamont, 1976). One half of those aged 31 to 35 had normal hearing and the proportion declined progressively, as follows: 41 to 50, 25 per cent; 56 to 60, 8 per cent; and 61 plus, 1 per cent. Nonetheless, because of the group's homogeneity, common interests, and long-term associations, "there is surprisingly good social adaptiveness . . . . It is easy for them to understand each other's conversations" (p. 260). Thus, as Heiner says, "It all depends."

Work and Career

Evidently the Swedish workers discussed in the foregoing section did not seek other kinds of employment after their hearing loss. However, many others must, as Andersson (1981) observes. "We are still in full possession of our mental faculties and our occupational skills, but are often forced to realize that they are no longer in demand" (p. 70).

The effects of hearing loss on employment vary. For example, one inquiry in France found that 50 per cent of deafened workers lost their jobs. Some remained with the same employer but earned lower salaries (Beuzart, 1981, p. 74). The 236 deafened respondents of Thomas and Gilhome-Herbst (1980) were significantly "less happy at work" than matched hearing controls (p. 81). Members of a Dutch hard of hearing organization were likely to do "lonely" work (Breed et al., 1981, p. 317). Of 56 deafened English workers, 23 per cent said that their jobs or job prospects had altered. A total of 41 per cent had experienced significant problems at work (Beattie, 1981, p. 17). Men excluded from social interaction at work were among the four groups Beattie cited as particularly vulnerable to the effects of hearing loss.

Two significant studies will be described here in greater detail. In the first study, Kyle and Wood (1983) interviewed 105 persons (51 per cent of their target population) identified through various agencies in the Avon area (near Bristol, England). Respondents were between 25 and 55 years of age, with onset of deafness during the previous ten years; with a hearing aid, 91 per cent could hear normal speech across a room (p. 35). Despite the relatively good hearing, 35 per cent felt that promotion at work was impossible (compared with 63 per cent of a prelingually deaf population and 16 per cent of hearing groups) (p. 55). The authors state that acquired hearing loss affects the quality of working life more than the level of earnings. Anxiety about the future was high (p. 58). When their deafness "became apparent," 39 per cent of the respondents informed their employer, but 37 per cent "never got around to" this; 95 per cent claimed that they could keep their jobs. To communicate, 93 per cent used a hearing aid;

16 per cent said that "often"—and 65 per cent, "sometimes"—they failed to understand instructions. Workmates were considered sympathetic or very sympathetic to loss of hearing by 53 per cent (p. 53).

The second study examined adults in Greater London of employment age with a hearing loss above 60 dB (Thomas, Lamont, and Harris, 1982). Of the 88 respondents, 68 were working; of these, 55 (81 per cent) said that their work had been affected by their poor hearing (pp. 39-40). The authors urge qualitative approaches as well as surveys, "because the diversity of problems encountered at work cannot be encompassed in a questionnaire" (p. 42). The diverse responses they list include the following: difficulty with the telephone, 75 per cent; difficulty coping with the public, 58 per cent; difficulty *doing* the job, 49 per cent; loss of promotion, 44 per cent; feeling left out, 38 per cent; difficulty with colleagues, 35 per cent; given less responsibility, 33 per cent; altered job assignment, 20 per cent; loss of job, 18 per cent; difficulties making friends at work, 16 per cent; felt little respect from workmates, 15 per cent; were demoted, 9 per cent (p. 41).

To summarize, the effects of hearing loss on employment are highly varied. The degree of loss and the nature of the job, particularly whether contact with the public and use of the phone are required, obviously affect the ability to perform the same job. Reduced interaction with colleagues is a common cause of dissatisfaction.

Family Life

The degree of family disruption is strongly linked with the degree of hearing loss and the age of onset. Several studies show that deafened persons have special difficulty with children. Beattie (1981) found that children, teenagers, and daughters of all ages were particularly impatient with deafened persons (p. 13). Noting that 50 per cent of male but only 16 per cent of female respondents felt that their poor hearing had affected their marriage, Beattie reasons that deafness requires a change in the husband's traditional role; accustomed to a dominant position, he has to become more dependent on his wife. Some 83 per cent of the men and 71 per cent of the women stated that family conversations were "often" or "sometimes" conducted without them. Older respondents living with two or more adults were especially affected by this exclusion. One third of the respondents felt that members of their families experienced stress when communicating with them (p. 13).

These findings are congruent with those of Kyle and Wood (1983). Of their 105 respondents, 86 per cent agreed that "deafness places a strain on hearing members of their families" and 43 per cent agreed that it means much less contact with relatives. However, 53 per cent stated that relatives and neighbors always tried to include a deaf person in their conversations (p. 48).

The Dutch hard of hearing adults indicated that contacts with their children demanded special effort; some children did not even want to go shopping with a deafened parent (Breed et al., 1981, p. 317).

In his experiment with simulated hearing loss, von der Lieth (1972) found that both he and his family became more irritable; indeed, he had to interrupt the one-week experiment twice because of family crises (p. 83). Warfield (1957) observed that her marriage began to deteriorate when she began openly to admit her hearing loss; earlier, her husband had supported her efforts to hide and deny it.

Social Interaction and Stigma

Certain attitudes and conduct of hearing people, as perceived by deafened persons, are summarized by Heider and Heider (1941): they are impatient with deaf persons' slowness to understand; they whisper about private matters in front of deaf people; they believe that since deaf people can't hear speech they can't understand and are therefore inferior; they pity the deaf; the deaf are overprotected by and lose their freedom to hearing people; hearing people slight and take advantage of the deaf; hearing people tease and make fun of the deaf; and hearing people misunderstand the deaf (pp. 81-96).

There is abundant evidence that hard of hearing and deaf persons *believe* they are stigmatized by hearing persons, but little evidence of the precise nature and degree of that stigma. In one study conducted in New York's Grand Central Station, four confederates approached persons randomly with cards stating that they were deaf and needed help to make a phone call; of those approached, 55 per cent agreed to help (Thayer, 1973, p. 9). In another study, 150 college students evaluated pictures and recordings of children, some of whom wore hearing aids and had "deaf or hard of hearing speech." Pictures were rotated randomly with recorded voices and judges were asked to evaluate the children for personality, intelligence, achievement, and appearance. Each speaker became "less attractive" with a hearing aid or deviant speech (Blood, Blood, and Danhauer, 1978).

How does impaired hearing affect personal interaction? The psychologist von der Lieth (1972), who simulated deafness, moved closer to speakers and unknowingly "violated their sense of personal space"; he remarked that "it was peculiar to see people withdraw when I approached them closely" (p. 84). A student engaging in a similar experiment noted that a clerk in a shop grew increasingly annoyed with his inability to understand. After he displayed a "hard of hearing" badge, the clerk became "kind but patronizing" (p. 85).

One social technique of some deafened people is to monopolize or dominate conversation to reduce the need to understand other speakers (Oyer and Oyer, 1979, p. 131). Harriet Martineau (1877), who used an ear trumpet, agreed: "One of the bad consequences of my deafness has been the making me far too much of a talker: and though friends whom I can trust aver that I am also a good listener, I certainly have never allowed a fair share of time and opportunity to slower and more modest and considerate speakers" (p. 216, Vol. 2). A psychologist writes that one of his patients "made outlandish bland attempts to bluff his way conversationally, answering questions by guesswork . . . trying to read lips, trying to control conversation, ignoring his flagrant contradictions, insisting his impairment 'never bothered' him" (Knapp, 1960a, p. 411).

A deafened woman gives the following account of her difficulties with group conversation:

> Often I will be with a group of people when suddenly I realize that I do not understand what they are talking about . . . . I sometimes ask people to repeat themselves . . . the time taken by one person to repeat the incident robs him or her of hearing the rest of the conversation . . . .this not only distracts and annoys people, but . . . disrupts the flow of conversation . . . . This is particularly true, I think, with humor . . . because so much of humor is spoken; a play upon words, a pun or quickly said punch line . . . . I can remember only too well pleading with someone to repeat a joke or story, only to have the person be evasive and say something like, "Oh, it was nothing much." (Scopaz, 1978, p. 12)

In one study, deafened subjects were asked what they did when they missed what was said. The most common answers were: asking for repetition, obtaining assistance from others, pretending or guessing, and doing nothing (Nett, 1960, p. 86).

The public stigma attached to hearing aids is often cited as a reason for not using them (Maurer and Rupp, 1979, p. 99). One deafened woman told her otologist she would "rather die" than wear a hearing aid. When she finally took a lipreading course, she kept the class a secret and did not give her professional name (Warfield, 1957).

Clearly, public attitudes and the beliefs of deafened individuals about them have profound effects. However, researchers have not adequately delineated the attitudes and conduct of different elements of the hearing public and the correct and incorrect beliefs of deafened people about these attitudes.

HEARING LOSS IN THE ELDERLY

Much of this review is applicable to adults of all ages. However, in some respects, elderly people have distinctive problems that should be considered separately, as has been done in several chapters in this book.

The prevalence of hearing loss increases dramatically with age, especially above 65 (Chapter 1, p. 13). Some observers believe that hearing loss can render the elderly "prime candidates for needless senility" (Maurer and Rupp, 1979, p. 97). It can also accentuate their social isolation, dependency, and loss of status (Beattie, 1981). Elderly people are less likely to join organizations for the hard of hearing, especially if they lost their hearing late in life (Miller, 1975, p. 62; Thomas and Gilhome-Herbst, 1980, p. 81).

Wax (1982) argues that elderly hearing-impaired persons suffer "double jeopardy" from two devalued conditions, that can produce "additive or cumulative effects" (p. 5). An example is the occurrence of depression as the most common psychiatric diagnosis both of deafened individuals (Knapp, 1960a; Ramsdell, 1970) and first admissions of elderly patients to hospitals (Zarit, 1980, p. 191).

Men are more vulnerable than women to the social and psychological impact of hearing loss and more likely to become overly dependent on others. Men, too, have been more likely to experience the trauma of retirement from work and the isolation that may accompany it; elderly deafened men may "find themselves virtually prisoners in solitary confinement" (Criswell, 1979, p. 36).

Four studies of the adjustment of deafened elderly persons have been reported. In the first study (Humphrey et al., 1981), 136 men and women over age 70, with a hearing loss greater than 35 dB (1000-2000-4000 Hz), were interviewed in London (p. 26). Only 21 per cent had hearing aids; 33 per cent were not aware that the National Health Service provided aids and 46 per cent did not know that they were entitled to free hearing services. Subjects were divided into four groups based on decibel loss. Those in Group A (N=36, mean dB loss 44) did not admit their hearing impairment. Group B (N=34, mean dB loss 52) members had never mentioned their hearing to a doctor, although 19 per cent felt "handicapped" by it; only 16 per cent had noted the loss before age 65. The individuals in Group C (N=37, mean dB loss 56) had seen a doctor but not been referred for a hearing aid; 26 per cent felt handicapped and 43 per cent had noted a loss before age 65. Those in Group D (N=30, mean dB loss 70) had seen doctors and been issued hearing aids; 62 per cent felt handicapped and 77 per cent were impaired before 65. Compared to Groups A, B, and C, Group D members were less likely to have a telephone or to listen to a radio and more likely to have fewer friends presently than in the past and to know about lipreading classes and clubs for hard of hearing people. The authors suggest that "the essentially social nature of the disability may discourage medical doctors from seeing it as a medical condition requiring attention" (p. 29).

The second study (Weinstein and Ventry, 1982) examined 80 male veterans age 65 or more (mean age 74) who were outpatients at a Veterans Administration medical center, with a mean hearing loss of 42 dB (500-1000-2000-3000 Hz) and a mean age of 68 at onset of hearing loss. One subjective and three objective tests of hearing loss, a 19-item scale assessing subjective social isolation, and a 38-item scale assessing objective social isolation were administered. The subjective measure of auditory loss correlated more highly with subjective and objective social isolation than did the three other auditory measures. Hearing loss, by all four measures, was significantly correlated with subjective social isolation.

In the third study (Thomas et al., 1983), data are presented on 239 volunteer participants in a longitudinal study of aging at the University of New Mexico Medical Center. While of great potential interest, it is disappointing because of deficiencies in the research design. For example, 20 participants were excluded from this analysis *because they wore hearing aids*, since the authors sought to evaluate the effects of *untreated* hearing deficits. Their criterion for "hearing impairment" was 16 decibels, and mean audiometric data for the group are not reported. Scores on the Speech Perception in Noise (SPIN) test (number correct of 50 words) ranged from 88 per cent for women ages 60 to 69 to 62 per cent for men 80 years of age and over; the pure tone average (PTA) threshold ranged from 8 dB for women ages 60 to 69 to 30 dB for women 80 years old and over. Subjects were advantaged socially, economically, and medically: 42 per cent had some college education; none had a major chronic illness or took prescription medication; 87 per cent of the men and 50 per cent of the women were married. Measures of anxiety, depression, and hostility were collected by self-administered questionnaire; measures of recall and subtraction were administered by an examiner. *No significant effects of hearing acuity were seen for psychological and social measures.* Correlations of .24 were found between recall and SPIN, and -.24 between subtraction scores and PTA ($p < .01$). The authors comment, "The question arises as to whether or not the impaired participants performed less well on the recall and subtraction subsections because they did not hear the questions adequately"! (p. 324).

Although this study has serious flaws, it reminds us of the wide range of hearing loss and of responses to it among elderly persons. Although national statistics lead us to expect that a significant proportion of almost any group of elderly persons will have impaired hearing, the adults in this study are not noticeably impaired. The authors recognize the "general good health and economic security" of their subjects. Despite their somewhat suspect findings on the relationship between hearing loss and cognitive deficit, Thomas and his coworkers conclude:

... many of the hearing impaired, healthy elderly adults in this study expressed anger and frustration at the tendency for others, including those providing services to older adults, to equate a hearing deficit with decreased functioning capability. It would seem that, at least for this group, hearing impairment is not synonymous with depression, isolation and confusion. (p. 324)

In the fourth study (Powers and Powers, 1978), 226 individuals aged 70 or older were interviewed in 1971. They represented all who could be reinterviewed from a random sample of 611 persons previously interviewed in 1960 in five Iowa counties (32 per cent of the 1960 group were known to have died by 1971). Asked, in 1960, if they had any difficulty hearing, 75 per cent said no; only 2 per cent reported a "significant" hearing problem. Of those with "nearly perfect" hearing in 1960, 98 per cent reported "nearly perfect" hearing in 1971 as well. Of the 51 persons who acknowledged some hearing difficulty in 1960, 23 (45 per cent) said their hearing had deteriorated; 39 per cent said it was the same; 2 per cent said that it had improved; and 14 per cent did not respond (p. 81).* When asked to list activities that gave them most satisfaction, how often they took trips, and how often they interacted with various relatives and friends, those with and without a hearing problem reported similar levels of interaction or satisfaction. Only one fifth of those with, compared to one third of those without, hearing difficulties indicated feelings of loneliness (p. 82).

Unfortunately the authors provide no information about the health, marital status, or living arrangements of their respondents, which might help to explain their surprising findings. Concerned that this study might misrepresent the extent of hearing loss among older persons, Hull (1978) wrote a strong letter to the editor of the journal in which it appeared. He

---

* Milne (1977) reports the responses of a random sample of 27,000 elderly Edinburgh residents to questions about hearing loss in the period 1968 to 1969 and in 1973; respondents were ages 62 to 90 during the first survey. Hearing loss of 112 men and 144 women in the period 1968 to 1969 was as follows (p. 13):

5-Year hearing loss	Men (%)	Women (%)
Deaf, 1968-1969, no change	19	15
Not deaf, 1968-1969, no change	34	54
Deaf, 1968-1969, worse later	31	14
Not deaf, 1968-1969, worse later	16	17

Far more showed an initial and subsequent hearing loss than the Iowa residents interviewed by Powers and Powers (1978). Were the measures of loss comparable? Were the survivors in the Iowa follow-up healthier? Does an urban-rural differential account for some of the differences?

argued that survey methods are unsuited to the self-report of hearing loss by elderly persons because of the probability of misunderstanding and because they are reluctant to admit a hearing loss and fear exploitation if they do.

Caution and Flexibility

In a study in which older and younger subjects were presented with a series of sounds within their range of hearing, older persons were likely to underreport sounds, suggesting that they were unwilling to "guess" (Rees and Botwinick, 1971). If this tendency applies to everyday situations—if older persons become cautious and less willing than the young to accept the minor risks of daily life—Zarit (1980) suggests that mild hearing loss could become needlessly disabling (p. 61).

Reduced flexibility evidently affects adaptability to hearing loss. Many elderly persons do not use a hearing aid if it is acquired after they are too old "to adapt and adjust to . . . the instrument" (Maurer and Rupp, 1979, p. 100). Arthritic fingers, decreased coordination, and a slowing of responses and movements can make inserting a hearing aid, adjusting the volume control, or changing the small battery difficult for many elderly persons (Chapter 6, page 87).

Nursing Home Residents

Burton (1981) surveyed 65 homes for the elderly in one region of England, asking which of 11 simple measures were taken for hearing-impaired residents. Only two measures—cleaning ear molds and examining ears for wax—were regularly carried out by more than half of the homes. "My observations suggest that patient handling processes in many of the 1,000 or so hospitals in the region . . . are likely to be very primitive indeed when it comes to assisting elderly patients with a hearing loss . . . " (p. 80).

The Prelingually Deaf Population

In contrast to the generally baneful effects of hearing loss among the elderly, a healthier view emerges of the elderly prelingual deaf (Becker, 1980; Meadow-Orlans and Orlans, 1983). Becker found the help and support of neighbors and friends central to the good adjustment of elderly members of an urban deaf community:

Individuals in this specially created society have used group membership to achieve a nonstigmatized personal identity and normalized social relationships. These factors stand them in good stead throughout the life cycle. It is when they become old, however, that these factors are especially useful in coping. (Becker, p. 98)

In a study of a similar, cohesive group in a New York apartment complex, Owens (1981) concluded that their "life satisfaction" was more closely related to informal than to formal or solitary activity (p. 57).

Elderly prelingually deaf persons constitute a distinct community with a lifetime of experience in accommodating to deafness. They do not necessarily welcome newly deafened persons of their age, nor do most of the latter wish to join their community or to form one of their own, as Kyle and Wood (1983) observe:

> ... there is little desire to be part of a community of hard of hearing people in those who become deaf. The idea that those with handicaps might benefit from personal contact with other people with the same problem is not considered to be of much relevance. In practice, it is just as easy to lipread or hear a hearing person as it is to have contact with someone else with acquired deafness. (p. 68)

While 84 per cent of respondents in their study expressed interest in learning to lipread, 98 per cent were not interested either in signing or in fingerspelling (p. 40).

A deafened Finnish man's comments about manual communication are pertinent:

> Traditionally manual communication methods have been the property of the deaf and if other aurally handicapped have wanted to use them it has been possible only under their auspices. It has meant, among other things, that manual communication must have been taken as a true language. If somebody has felt that he needs visual cues in communication he has been obliged to learn them as a whole system and exactly in the "right" form. Often this requirement has discouraged hard of hearing and even deafened people from learning any visual marks at all. (Suomela, 1981, p. 88)

These remarks reflect personal experience, not systematic research. Nevertheless they tap a familiar attitude—both a cause and an effect of the prelingually deaf community's cohesiveness—which helps to explain its members' relatively effective adjustment to aging.

CONCLUSION

Although this chapter has focused on the problems and difficulties of hearing loss in adulthood, in no way does that minimize or devalue the positive adjustment, intelligence, stamina, and courage exhibited by count-less deafened individuals. In the personal documents examined, these qualities were demonstrated many times. One way of viewing responses to this sensory deprivation is to marvel at the adaptability and determination demonstrated by so many persons. The personal documents also affirm the anguish, frustration, anger, anxiety, and grief at removal from the accustomed world of sound and speech.

The many studies reviewed here have demonstrated, although they did not fully analyze and describe, the widely varied responses to adult hearing loss (see also Orlans and Meadow-Orlans, 1985). The difference between the "bridge of sighs" and the "stepping-stones of self-determination" depends on many things, most obviously including—yet often overlooked—the severity of the impairment. Hearing muffled speech is very different from hearing no speech at all. Thus, researchers who gloss over the residual hearing of their "deaf" subjects and report no observable or "testable" social-psychological consequences of impaired hearing serve neither social science nor social service adequately. Deafened people can learn, and can be helped, to cope; but obliviousness to the different effects of different degrees of hearing loss does not further that goal.

The reports of a heightened tendency to paranoia are mixed and conflicting. Despite the widespread belief in this reaction, the evidence is contradictory. Evidence of depression is more consistent, possibly because the term is used both in professional diagnosis and in everyday speech. Withdrawal, loneliness, isolation, nervousness, and fatigue all seem well documented as frequent concomitants of the deafened condition.

The impact of deafness on work life depends on the nature of the work and the need to use the telephone and converse with people. Sociable relations with workmates are commonly disturbed. The manifold effects on family life depend on the nature of previous relationships, the age at which hearing loss occurs, and the spouse's readiness to serve as an intermediary and aide.

Elderly persons who live in the community have very different responses and needs than those in retirement or nursing homes. Further investigation is needed into the effects of noise and the urban environment on hearing-impaired elderly people. A comparison of the deafened elderly with elderly prelingual deaf groups provides another example of the importance of a supportive family and friends for a good adjustment.

The attitudes and conduct of hearing persons are obviously important to the adjustment of those with a hearing loss and deserve far more study than they have received. So do the reasons for, and precise nature of, the negative attitudes toward deafened persons and the frequent reluctance of the hearing-impaired elderly to admit a hearing loss or to wear a hearing aid, compared, for example, with the more ready acceptance of glasses for visual impairment.

This review has raised as many questions as it has answered. The questions are intriguing and the answers important if we are to understand better and to improve the lives of deafened people.

REFERENCES

Alpiner, J. G., Chevrette, W., Glascoe, G., Metz, M., and Olsen, B. (1974). *The Denver Scale of Communication Function.* Unpublished manuscript, University of Denver.

Andersson, B. (1981). On becoming and being a deafened adult. In H. Hartmann (Ed.), *Congress report* (pp. 70-73). Hamburg: First International Congress of the Hard of Hearing, Deutscher Schwerhörigenbund.

Barker, R. G., and Wright, B. A. (1952). The social psychology of adjustment to physical disability. In J. F. Garrett (Ed.), *Psychological aspects of physical disability* (Rehabilitation Service Series No. 210, pp. 18-32). Washington, DC: Office of Vocational Rehabilitation.

Barker, R. G., in collaboration with B. A. Wright, L. Meyerson, and M. R. Gonick (1953). *Adjustment to physical handicap and illness: A survey of the social psychology of physique and disability.* New York: Social Science Research Council Bulletin 55 (rev.).

Beattie, J. A. (1981). *Social aspects of acquired hearing loss in adults.* A report on the research project funded by the Department of Health and Social Security and carried out in the Postgraduate School of Applied Social Studies, University of Bradford (England), 1978-1981: Summary of Contents and Findings.

Becker, G. (1980). *Growing old in silence.* Berkeley: University of California Press.

Beuzart, E. (1981). Consequences of a hearing loss acquired during professional activity. In H. Hartmann (Ed.), *Congress report* (pp. 74-76). Hamburg: First International Congress of the Hard of Hearing, Deutscher Schwerhörigenbund.

Blood, G. W., Blood, I. M., and Danhauer, J. L. (1978). Listeners' impressions of normal-hearing and hearing-impaired children. *Journal of Communication Disorders, 11,* 513-518.

Breed, P. C. M., van den Horst, A. P. J. M., Mous, T. J. M. (1981). Psychosocial problems in suddenly deafened adolescents and adults. In H. Hartmann (Ed.), *Congress report* (pp. 313-320). Hamburg: First International Congress of the Hard of Hearing, Deutscher Schwerhörigenbund.

Brooks, D. N. (1979). Counselling and its effects on hearing aid use. *Scandinavian Audiology, 8,* 101-107.

Burton, D. K. (1981). Hearing loss among the elderly. In H. Hartmann (Ed.), *Congress report* (pp. 77-81). Hamburg: First International Congress of the Hard of Hearing, Deutscher Schwerhörigenbund.

Cooper, A. F., Kay, D. W. K., Curry, A. R., Garside, R. F., and Roth, M. (1974). Hearing loss in paranoid and affective psychosis of the elderly. *Lancet, 2,* 851-854.

Criswell, E. C. (1979). Deaf Action Center's senior citizen program. *Journal of Rehabilitation of the Deaf, 12,* 36-40.

Diamant, H. (1976). Social handicap among workers with noise-induced hearing loss. *Acta Otolaryngologica, 81,* 260-263.

Elliott, H. (1978). *Acquired deafness—Shifting gears.* Unpublished manuscript.

Ewertsen, H. W., and Birk-Nielsen, H. (1973). Social hearing handicap index. *Audiology, 12,* 180-187.

Giolas, T. G. (1982). *Hearing-handicapped adults.* Englewood Cliffs, NJ: Prentice-Hall.

Giolas, T. G., Owens, E., Lamb, S. H., and Schubert, E. D. (1979). Hearing performance inventory. *Journal of Speech and Hearing Disorders, 44,* 169-195.

Glasgow, E. (1954). *The woman within.* New York: Harcourt, Brace.

Heider, F., and Heider, G. M. (1941). Studies in the psychology of the deaf (No. 2). *Psychological Monographs, 53* (Whole No. 242).

Heiner, M. H. (1949) *Hearing is believing.* Cleveland: World Publishing.

High, W. S., Fairbanks, G., and Glorig, A. (1964). Scale of self-assessment of hearing handicap. *Journal of Speech and Hearing Disorders, 29*, 215-230.

Hull, R. H. (1978). The powers to misrepresent. *ASHA, 20,* 462-463.

Humphrey, C., Gilhome-Herbst, K., and Faurqi, S. (1981). Some characteristics of the hearing-impaired elderly who do not present themselves for rehabilitation. *British Journal of Audiology, 15,* 25-30.

Hunter, C. C. (1978). *A pilot study of late deafened adults.* Master's thesis. California State University, Northridge.

Kay, D. W. K., Cooper, A. F., Garside, R. F., and Roth, M. (1976). The differentiation of paranoid from affective psychoses by patients' premorbid characteristics. *British Journal of Psychiatry, 129*, 207-215.

Knapp, P. H. (1960a). Emotional aspects of hearing loss. In D. A. Barbara (Ed.), *Psychological and psychiatric aspects of speech and hearing* (pp. 396-439). Springfield, IL: Charles C Thomas. (Reprinted from *Psychosomatic Medicine,* 1948, *X*)

Knapp, P. H. (1960b). The ear, listening and hearing. In D. A. Barbara (Ed.), *Psychological and psychiatric aspects of speech and hearing* (pp. 92-109). Springfield, IL: Charles C Thomas. (Reprinted from the *Journal of the American Psychoanalytic Association,* 1953, *1*)

Kyle, J. G., and Wood, P. L. (1983). *Social and vocational aspects of acquired hearing loss.* Final report to MSC, School of Education Research Unit, University of Bristol.

Luey, H. S. (1980). Between worlds: The problems of deafened adults. *Social Work in Health Care, 5,* 253-265.

Martineau, H. (1983). *Autobiography.* London: Virago Press. (First published in 1877.)

Maurer, J. F. (1976). *Working with the elderly.* Washington, DC: The National Council on Aging.

Maurer, J. F., and Rupp, R. R. (1979). *Hearing and aging: Tactics for intervention.* New York: Grune and Stratton.

McCartney, B. (1981). The psychology of the hard of hearing—which world do I belong in? In H. Hartmann (Ed.), *Congress report* (pp. 12-26). Hamburg: First International Congress of the Hard of Hearing, Deutscher Schwerhörigenbund.

Meadow, K. P. (1980). *Deafness and child development.* Berkeley: University of California Press.

Meadow-Orlans, K. P., and Orlans, H. (1983, July). *Mental health status and needs of deafened adults.* Paper presented at the Congress of the World Federation of the Deaf, Palermo, Italy.

Menninger, K. A. (1952). Psychiatric aspects of physical disability. In J. F. Garrett (Ed.), *Psychological aspects of physical disability* (Rehabilitation Service Series No. 210, pp. 8-17). Washington, DC: Office of Vocational Rehabilitation.

Miller, L. V. (1975). The adult and the elderly: Health care and hearing loss. *Volta Review, 77,* 57-63.

Milne, J. S. (1977). A longitudinal study of hearing loss in older people. *British Journal of Audiology, 11,* 7-14.

Mulrooney, J. (1973, October). The newly-deafened adult. In *Proceedings,* National Conference on Program Development for and with Deaf People (pp. 40-43).

Sponsored by the Office of Public Service, Gallaudet College, and Cooperative Extension, University of Maryland, Washington, DC.

Myklebust, H. R. (1964). *The psychology of deafness.* New York: Grune and Stratton.

Nett, E. M. (1960). *The relationships between audiological measures and handicap.* A project of the University of Pittsburgh School of Medicine and the Office of Vocational Rehabilitation, U.S. Department of Health, Education, and Welfare.

Noble, W. G., and Atherly, G. R. C. (1970). The hearing measure scale: A questionnaire for the assessment of auditory disability. *Journal of Auditory Research, 10,* 229-250.

Orlans, H., and Meadow-Orlans, K. P. (1985, January/February). Responses to hearing loss: Effects on social life, leisure, and work. *Shhh, 6*(1), 4-7.

Owens, D. J. (1981). *The relationship of frequency and types of activity to life satisfaction in elderly deaf people.* Unpublished doctoral dissertation, School of Education, Health and Nursing Arts, New York University.

Oyer, H. J., and Oyer, E. J. (1979). Social consequences of hearing loss for the elderly. *Allied Health and Behavioral Sciences, 2,* 123-137.

Powers, J. K., and Powers, E. A. (1978). Hearing problems of elderly persons: Social consequences and prevalence. *ASHA, 20,* 79-83.

Ramsdell, D. A. (1970). The psychology of the hard of hearing and the deafened adult. In H. Davis and S. R. Silverman (Eds.), *Hearing and deafness* (3rd ed.)(pp. 435-446). New York: Holt, Rinehart and Winston.

Rees, J., and Botwinick, J. (1971). Detection and decision factors in auditory behavior of the elderly. *Journal of Gerontology, 26,* 133-136.

Reichstein, J., and von der Lieth, L. (1981). Learning from the experiences of student teachers with simulated hearing loss. In H. Hartmann (Ed.), *Congress report* (pp. 302-307). Hamburg: First International Congress of the Hard of Hearing, Deutscher Schwerhörigenbund.

Rosen, J. K. (1979). Psychological and social aspects of the evaluation of acquired hearing impairment. *Audiology, 18,* 238-252.

Rousey, C. L. (1971). Psychological reactions to hearing loss. *Journal of Speech and Hearing Disorders, 36,* 382-389.

Schein, J. D. (1968). *The deaf community.* Washington, DC: Gallaudet College Press.

Schein, J. D., and Delk, M. T., Jr. (1974). *The deaf population of the United States.* Silver Spring, MD: National Association of the Deaf.

Schein, J. D., Gentile, A., and Haase, K. W. (1970, April). *Development and evaluation of an expanded hearing loss scale questionnaire* (Vital and Health Statistics, Series 2, No. 37). National Center for Health Statistics. Washington, DC: U.S. Government Printing Office.

Scopaz, V. M. (1978). Living with a hearing loss. *Hearing Rehabilitation Quarterly, 3,* 11-13.

Solomon, M. (1977). *Beethoven.* New York: Schirmer Books.

Stephens, S. D. G. (1980). Evaluating the problems of the hearing impaired. *Audiology, 19,* 205-220.

Suomela, E. K. (1981). Identification problems of deafened persons and communication: Some suggestions. In H. Hartmann (Ed.), *Congress report* (pp. 87-92). Hamburg: First International Congress of the Hard of Hearing, Deutscher Schwerhörigenbund.

Thayer, S. (1973). Lend me your ears: Racial and sexual factors in helping the deaf. *Journal of Personality and Social Psychology, 28*, 8-11.

Thomas, A. J. (1981). Acquired deafness and mental health. *British Journal of Medical Psychology, 54*, 219-229.

Thomas, A., and Gilhome-Herbst, K. (1980). Social and psychological implications of acquired deafness for adults of employment age. *British Journal of Audiology, 14*, 76-85.

Thomas, A., Lamont, M., and Harris, M. (1982). Problems encountered at work by people with severe acquired hearing loss. *British Journal of Audiology, 16*, 39-43.

Thomas, P. D., Hunt, W. C., Garry, P. J., Hood, R. B., Goodwin, J. M., and Goodwin, J. S. (1983). Hearing acuity in a healthy elderly population: effects of emotional, cognitive, and social status. *Journal of Gerontology, 38*, 321-325.

Trybus, R. J. (1983, July). *Hearing impaired patients in public psychiatric hospitals throughout the United States.* Paper presented at the Congress of the World Federation of the Deaf, Palermo, Italy.

Ventry, I. M., and Weinstein, B. E. (1982). The hearing handicap inventory for the elderly: A new tool. *Ear and Hearing, 3*, 128-134.

von der Lieth, L. (1972). Experimental social deafness. *Scandinavian Audiology, 1*, 81-87.

Warfield, F. (1957). *Keep listening.* New York: Viking Press.

Wax, T. (1982). The hearing impaired aged: Double jeopardy or double challenge. *Gallaudet Today, 12*, 3-7.

Weinstein, B. E., and Ventry, I. M. (1982). Hearing impairment and social isolation in the elderly. *Journal of Speech and Hearing Research, 25*, 593-599.

Zarit, S. H. (1980). *Aging and mental disorders, psychological approaches to assessment and treatment.* New York: The Free Press.

Zarnoch, J. M., and Alpiner, J. G. (1976). *The Denver Scale of Communication Function for Senior Citizens Living in Retirement Centers.* University of Denver.

Chapter 4
A Personal Account

Jack Ashley

Before I suddenly lost my hearing completely 16 years ago, I had given very little thought to the problems of deafness. My much loved mother was hard of hearing in her later years but it was more of a nuisance than a tragedy. The family had to raise their voices for her and sometimes repeat things, but the greatest difficulty was to persuade her to wear a hearing aid. When she eventually did so, the difficulties were not wholly resolved but they were greatly eased. Clarity of speech and the avoidance of background clatter or obtrusive music enabled her to cope adequately.

The difficulties of very severe hearing loss impinged on my consciousness in only one minor respect. In my adolescence, I knew the father of one of my friends had very great difficulty in hearing speech unless people shouted clearly to him. He was too poor to pay for any kind of hearing aid, and in those early days they were not freely available, as they were later, because Britain's splendid National Health Service was not then in effect.

When any group of friends visited the house and chatted together, an occasional point would be explained to my friend's father by one of his family and he sometimes made a comment; he was a thoughtful and highly intelligent man. As the conversation developed, topics would change from one to another. The deaf father would, after reflection, make a further comment on the subject we had left some time ago. This was always disconcerting and, after a slight pause, we would assent to his view with nods of agreement—for he was a friendly man. We would then resume our conversation, conscious that, although he was with us, he was unable to follow the discussion. We accepted this as a natural concomitant of his deafness.

Without rancor, indeed even with good will, we took it for granted as the natural order of things that, because of his deafness, he could not participate in our discussions except for his occasional forays. We accepted these patiently, as an understandable interruption, before proceeding with the natural progression of our conversation. Our youthful ignorance and selfishness make me blanch in retrospect.

This was the sum total of my experience of, and interest in, deafness. The thunderbolt of sudden, total loss of hearing 16 years ago was, therefore, all the more devastating.

THE THUNDERBOLT OF DEAFNESS

I was unprepared for deafness. I had no experience of its effect. I was completely unaware of its profound and far-reaching consequences on my life and on my family. It was shattering beyond belief.

On one day I could hear fairly well, the only impediment being a perforated eardrum. A few weeks later, after a disastrous operation to repair the eardrum, I was virtually totally deaf. The plunge from a normally hearing world into one of almost total silence meant the plummeting of my happiness, aspirations, and hopes for the future.

Over the next few tortured months, during which a very slight modicum of hearing remained, trembling in the balance, delicately protecting me from the brink of despair, I learned the fundamental difference between a hearing person and one who is very profoundly deaf. It was, it seemed to me then, the difference between living life to the full and merely existing in misery.

Apart from the traumatic shock of this change, I felt a profound sense of loss. The truism that there is no point in worrying about what might have been offers no consolation to the suddenly deafened person. I was aware that my life had undergone a profound and appalling change. I knew that the confident, easygoing relationships with people, which I had always taken for granted, had gone forever. I felt sure that every personal encounter, friendly or not, from now on would be fraught with difficulty. My political ambitions had been demolished at a stroke. Overnight I had been transformed from an eager, aspiring MP, tipped by some as a "high flyer" destined for Ministerial office, to a disabled person whose political hopes lay in ruins.

It seemed that there was no hope of remaining as a Member of Parliament. The requirements of that honorable but testing profession were to listen, converse, argue, and debate. I had to engage in dialogue with constituents and participate in the exchanges at Westminster. A representative who is unable to listen to representations, or to hear the responses from Ministers when he makes them, hardly qualifies for that job. Hearing is more crucial to the task of being an MP than to almost any other profession.

Yet, even during that traumatic period, I never quite gave up hope. There were three reasons. First, I was determined to utilize the fragment of hearing that remained and fight on regardless. Second, I decided to communicate by lipreading and master the art as soon as humanly possible.

Third, my wife sustained and encouraged me with extraordinary determination, loyalty, and faith. Her belief was that the vital requirements for a Parliamentarian were judgment, political skill, and experience. She argued that none of these was impaired by my deafness. I embarked immediately on the task of learning to lipread.

The remnant of hearing left was so miniscule that it scarcely registered on an audiogram chart. Perhaps 1 per cent remained. Yet it greatly helped my efforts at lipreading. Even in those early traumatic months, by using a hearing aid and concentrating with ferocious intensity, I could stumble along with a conversation. That tiny, imperceptible fragment of hearing had a remarkably disproportionate effect on my capacity to lipread, shocked and exhausted as I was. At that time I had no idea of its tremendous significance.

It was only a few months later that the wisp of hearing vanished. Then I appreciated the difference between the very hard of hearing and the totally deaf. People had been remarking on the remarkable grasp of lipreading I had acquired within weeks. In fact it was because the modicum of hearing enabled me to understand to some extent the sounds that are the most difficult to lipread. It helped me to keep in tenuous touch with the hearing world and, no doubt, it had a helpful psychological effect; but its crucial importance was that it was a vital adjunct to lipreading.

Those who are hard of hearing face serious difficulties, which depend on the extent of their hearing loss and their attitude toward it; totally deaf persons face problems of an entirely different order of magnitude. Yet the public use the word "deafness" as an umbrella term to cover all forms of hearing loss. No wonder deaf people are bedeviled by being misunderstood.

My experiences are naturally different from those who were born deaf, because I have made the bleak journey from the world of hearing to the world of silence. The born deaf are denied the advantages gained by the deafened before their hearing loss, yet they are spared the desolating sense of loss. I had enjoyed the natural acquisition of speech and language and had a knowledge of the hearing world. These are priceless assets in attempting to cope with total deafness. But I was painfully and permanently aware of what I had lost. My perception of that loss is a lifelong burden.

The emotional response of any individual to deafness is a very personal matter, determined by his or her temperament and expectations as well as the degree of deafness. However, it is also affected by the practical experiences of coping with deafness and how well or badly these turn out.

My own experiences are in some ways different from those of anyone else, insofar as I understand that I am the only totally deaf person in the world who is an elected member of a legislative assembly. The nature of the problems that consequently arise are probably unique. Yet, underlying these distinctive features lies the reality that all totally deaf people face similar problems that are an inevitable product of this particular disability.

The essential difference of my experience lies in holding public office. This, paradoxically, compounds the problems of deafness immeasurably and simultaneously makes them easier.

IN A MAELSTROM OF SPEECH

Any totally deaf person, skilled or unskilled, who works alone or in an environment that minimizes the need for difficult communication, minimizes the problems caused by his disability. Conversely, being a Member of the British Parliament or any other legislature must maximize them. It was in a maelstrom of the spoken word that I chose to remain after losing my hearing, a place in which no one else suffered grievous hearing loss, in which no sign language was used, in which there were no interpreters, and which was the most public of all places.

To complicate a complicated matter even further, I chose to return alone. I could understand my wife, even in those early days, because she spoke with such consideration and clarity, but she had family responsibilities with our three daughters; also, I wanted to assert my independence in Parliament. Hence, I found myself encompassed in an extraordinary invisible glass cage while carrying out my Parliamentary duties. It was a remarkable experience.

Before I attempted to resume my Parliamentary duties, I needed the support of the people I represented, and some knowledge of lipreading was necessary. The support was readily, even warmly, forthcoming, and people seemed far more confident than I was that I could carry on as a Member of Parliament. Either they did not appreciate the magnitude of the problem or they had a touching faith in my ability to cope. Whatever the reason, the support was there in rich abundance.

Acquiring skill in lipreading is not, of course, something that can be done overnight. I had the imaginative help of my wife, who devised her own version of learning vowels and consonants by eye, and various friends were willing to assist in any way possible. However, even with this help and with intense, sustained concentration, I found that progress was depressingly slow.

Naturally I encountered all the usual problems of learning this difficult means of communication. Nevertheless, it was a vital lifeline for me. I had to clutch it and improve my hold on it as swiftly as possible. Even today, after much experience, I would not rank myself among the best of lipreaders, but, at that time, I was quite a poor one. Yet the choice was stark—return or resign. I had to go back, despite my inadequate standard of lipreading, or go elsewhere. I chose to go back. It was in Parliament, and in the constituency I represent, at public functions as well as in private discussions, that I had to make my mistakes, learn my lessons, and somehow make it work.

The task was not as daunting as I expected in my constituency; one reason for this was that my wife usually accompanied me. Heaven help the deafened person who is alone. Without my wife I would have survived, but without her I could not have remained an MP.

It was at those vital political meetings in my constituency, where I was to report on political issues and answer questions, that she took notes to supplement my lipreading. She caught the fine nuances of voice inflection that I could no longer hear and reflected them in her notes in addition to the main points of discussion. Thus, by this combination of rudimentary lipreading and my wife's notes, I was able to reestablish the essential contact with my political base.

Similarly, at my Advice Bureaus we worked together and managed without any of the monumental problems we at first envisaged. Today my wife's notes are an adjunct to my lipreading when I talk to my constituents at Advice Bureaus, but in those early years my lipreading was an adjunct to her notes. Yet, by whatever means, the essential point was that I was communicating with my local political party and my constituents. That was really all that mattered. Once communication was established I was able to fulfill my role as a Member of Parliament and apply my political judgment, knowledge, and experience to carry out my duties.

If the cooperation of my wife was vital, the attitude of my constituents was remarkable. Few, if any of them, had had any experience of deafness. In the early days, many were only vaguely aware that I was deaf; some probably thought that I was hard of hearing. However, when my constituents met me they accepted my total deafness and without further ado got on with the business in hand. It did not matter whether they came for advice or help from me, or whether they came to express their political views on the issues of the day; they made their approach to their Member of Parliament and I understood them. Perhaps unwittingly, they helped to restore my confidence and give me enormous encouragement.

It is, however, one thing to establish and secure a political base in a city when one is suddenly and totally deafened, and another to participate alone in Parliament. A Member of Parliament naturally has some status in his constituency, but at Westminster he is only one of 650. It was there, where all are MPs, that the major challenge lay, and where I had to take stock, reassess my new role, and adapt if possible.

The first thing I had to do was recognize reality and face the fact that I could no longer aspire to the great offices of state. This is the understandable ambition of all MPs, because it is with Ministers that real power resides. Membership of Parliament is a prerequisite to Ministerial office and office is the reward of successful Members.

I was then Parliamentary Private Secretary to the Deputy Prime Minister. A PPS is a kind of right-hand man in a position usually regarded as the first stepping stone to becoming a Minister. Immediately after I became deaf, I offered the Deputy Prime Minister my resignation, but he refused to accept it. However, a few months later, he was appointed Foreign Secretary and, this time, when I pressed my resignation, he had no alternative but to accept. Being the Parliamentary Private Secretary to a Minister with such a demanding job could not be carried out with the necessary efficiency and diplomacy by someone groping in a fog of silence.

There was an interesting difference in the attitude of Members of Parliament compared with that of constituents. The MPs, on all sides, were friendly enough, yet there was an obvious wariness about some of them. They wanted to help but were not certain how to do so. Some were willing to cooperate but unwilling to initiate. If I approached them they would always respond, but sometimes their response was no more than adequate and that would be the end of the matter. I was perceiving for the first time the polite but restrained reaction of colleagues who had no wish to wound but no wish to help. There was a fear of being involved. This was a natural reaction that will be recognized by any deaf person who has ventured across generally accepted business or social barriers.

A totally deaf person in Parliament is left in no doubt of the limitations on some relationships imposed by his disability. I once said that I lost none of my friends when I became deaf, but it was not until I became deaf that I knew who *were* my friends. All my experience since has confirmed that judgment. The only conceivable response from me was to accept any indifference and recognize that it was one of the unhappy and unavoidable consequences of deafness.

Fortunately, I found a significant number of MPs willing to help. They were not always the ones I expected. A few of those who had earlier been friendly showed a disinclination to deal with the difficulties, whereas apparently dour personalities were surprisingly willing to do whatever they could. They would speak more slowly and clearly, make sure I had understood some particularly important point in a group discussion, or slip into the next seat to me and offer to take notes. Basic human qualities are put to the test when a person has to react to a disabled colleague. Deafness gave me a new insight into the qualities of other MPs and I adjusted my reaction to them accordingly.

However, my relationships with Parliamentary colleagues were much more complex than merely reacting to friendly approaches or calculated indifference. The question of my independence was vital and I had to retain my freedom to hit hard on the political issues of the day, regardless of whether my opponents had shown personal understanding of deafness.

This decision is not as simple or obvious as it may appear. If I have been in difficulty at a meeting or an informal discussion and a political opponent takes the trouble to write a helpful note, there is a natural and instinctive tendency to be appreciative; but gratitude is a false basis on which to build political relationships. I could not allow deafness, or any of its consequences, to affect my political attitudes, for this would have destroyed me as a politician.

CHOOSING POLITICAL ISSUES

Being totally deaf in Parliament meant facing unique questions on the choice of political issues. One of the most important was how far I should specialize in helping disabled people, including the deaf. Obviously, I would be asked by disabled people to make representations for them, and being disabled myself meant that I would have a deeper understanding of their problems. There was always the risk that a disabled MP campaigning for disabled people could be misunderstood. Perhaps my best contribution would be to show that despite the disability of total deafness I could still be a normal MP campaigning on a wide range of issues.

I decided to stay on the wider issues but to include disablement as an important subject. This part of my work expanded, and I soon became Chairman of the Parliamentary All Party Disablement Group, an influential pressure group making representations to the Government and initiating new legislation.

When I reassessed my role, I found that abandoning the climb up the Ministerial ladder gave me freedom to pursue any issues that interested me and to campaign on them. It is a privilege of MPs to highlight issues and focus Parliamentary and public opinion on them. The first major issue that I took up after losing my hearing was the fight for compensation to thalidomide-damaged children. This became a national—indeed an international— scandal when the company that marketed the drug denied liability and refused to pay compensation. The British *Sunday Times* led the battle outside Parliament and I led it inside. I was privileged to open a full Parliamentary debate on the subject, speaking at the Despatch box directly opposite the Secretary of State for Health, who was to reply for the Government.

After that campaign, which lasted many months, I took up others covering a wide range of issues. These included the need for a Royal Commission on legal procedures, a network of sanctuaries for battered wives, compensation for adverse medical drug reactions, reform of the law on rape to give victims more legal protection in court, and a code of conduct guiding drug exports to Third World countries. In some cases success was complete. The Royal Commission was established after a campaign that lasted less than two months; many sanctuaries for victims of family violence were set up; and the law on rape was reformed.

Many of the issues that I took up related to disabled people. I was actively involved as a sponsor of Britain's first piece of comprehensive legislation to give disabled people new rights. I also pursued subjects of special interest to deaf people.

For example, Britain's research into deafness was slight and sporadic and I proposed an Institute of Hearing Research. The officials at the Department of Health were adamantly opposed, largely on grounds of cost, but it was set up in 1977. It is now a well-established, flourishing institution carrying out valuable research.

Another main issue affecting deaf people was the phasing out by the Government of the technically proficient but cumbersome body-worn hearing aid available to deaf people under the National Health Service, and replacement with a modern, behind-the-ear aid. Today, every deaf person in Britain can have a free ear-level hearing aid, as well as free service and batteries.

MANAGING THE MEDIA AND PARLIAMENTARY DEBATE

I have been surprised by how little total deafness has handicapped me in conducting these campaigns. By using all the Parliamentary tools available, and by the use of publicity to win public support, I have achieved my aims as effectively as any other MP. The media present no serious problems which cannot be overcome. On television, as I know the subject matter and discuss the general ground with the interviewer before going before the cameras and bright lights, I manage quite well. My training as a television producer is helpful while I am in the studio. I am familiar with the atmosphere, know how everything works, and enjoy the challenge.

Radio interviews are less tense than television. There are no bright lights and fewer diversions during interviews. I often do radio interviews by telephone; these are easiest of all, because my wife has perfected a system of listening to the interviewer's incoming questions on an earpiece extension and silently repeating the words for me to lipread as soon as they are spoken. This system, which we have used for countless live national radio programs, is very successful. My secretary uses it also; my daily routine, like that of all politicians, includes many telephone calls; yet my deafness causes no problems.

The use of the media is also helpful in keeping me in touch with my constituency. The very good newspaper and radio station in Stoke-on-Trent, the city which I represent, keeps my constituents informed of all my Parliamentary activities.

The media coverage has been of crucial importance before and during General Elections. I have fought five elections since I lost my hearing. Inevitably, I wondered about the public's reaction to deafness. Would there be any prejudice? Would people be prepared to turn out and vote?

The first election campaign was the most dramatic of all because of the timing. By pure chance, the election was called during the holiday weeks in my constituency, which has a long tradition of local industry closing down for two special weeks. Practically everyone takes their holidays at this time, and there is an exodus from the city to seaside resorts. I was fighting the election campaign not only without hearing but also without voters. However, it all turned out well in the end, and I was elected with a comfortable majority.

Over the years I have benefited from the cumulative effect of my work. My activities have brought me into close touch with many of my constituents. Through the media exposure they know me as a person, not as a remote Parliamentarian. I have helped many of them, met them at my Advice Bureaus or when presenting prizes at their school or crowning their festival queens. Their continued acceptance of my deafness, and their warm response to me, has been one of the most heartening aspects of my political career.

In Parliament it has been slightly different. The pace of life is inevitably faster and more demanding and the whole place throbs with activity. Without my hearing, even those experiences that others find relaxing, such as chatting on the terraces on a summer evening between votes, are a strain because of lipreading.

Nevertheless, the attitude of MPs to deafness has improved over the years. There are still some lonely moments—and some still don't want to know—but the general attitude is friendly and helpful. I saw this strikingly illustrated a few months ago when I was a member of a British Parliamentary delegation to an international conference in Nairobi. The conference hall was so huge that it was difficult to see the expressions on people's faces, let alone lipread. The other ten MPs on the delegation—most of whom were my political opponents—took turns all week to take notes for me. It was a remarkable collective endeavor.

One of the greatest political honors I have received, and something of great practical value to me as a totally deaf MP, has been my appointment as a Privy Councillor. This is an honor always given to Cabinet Ministers, occasionally to middle ranking Ministers, and very rarely to back benchers. Its practical effect is that I am now, by virtue of being a Privy Councillor, called early in debates when I want to participate. (Those who preside over our debates [called Speakers] were in the past very considerate to me, but they had to keep to the rules of the debate.) It is significant for me because it reduces fatigue as I do not have to concentrate on a large number of preceding speeches.

A most important change has been in the way that I follow the spoken word. For nine years I had to rely upon lipreading and the notes of busy MPs to understand what was going on in Parliament. This was supplemented by reading the following day's verbatim report of the proceedings. Obviously, I had to prepare very carefully before intervening, and my effectiveness in the cut and thrust of debate was diminished. There was a limit to the risks that could be taken.

The new method was originated seven years ago when my wife sought a system to enable me to follow Parliamentary proceedings with less strain. She suggested linking Palantype, a form of mechanized shorthand, to a visual display unit. After some university research, the system was developed and I used it in Parliament.

It proved to be a great boon. I could follow all the proceedings without difficulty, even though the phonetics, and occasional operator errors caused by fast speech, required concentration. Recently, a modernized model was demonstrated in London, which has an accuracy rate of 95 per cent, compared with the present equipment's accuracy rate of 71 per cent. This is dramatic progress which will not only help me, but will eventually help many other deaf people.

These examples may give some idea of the special difficulties I encountered in Parliament and some of the means I adopted to overcome them. Unexpectedly, being in public life made deafness easier for me to cope with, because as a result of becoming well known as an MP, through news coverage, programs like "This Is Your Life," and documentaries in connection with my work, the public developed a friendly relationship with me and became more sympathetic to my deafness. For example, railway porters and taxi drivers often go to great lengths to speak clearly for me.

WALKING TALL

Although not as monumental as I expected, the problems due to deafness were real enough. So few people understand the profundity of total deafness and the difficulty of lipreading strangers—especially if they merely raise their voices and speak quickly—that when they approach me for a chat about my latest campaign and I cannot follow them, they become embarrassed. I then have to decide whether simply to shrug the whole thing off with a casual and friendly word or to start reassuring them, bringing out paper and pen, and clarifying the issues.

Helping deaf people, and attempting to communicate with them, is a laudable endeavor. It must, nevertheless, be carefully watched because it can so easily become patronizing. It is not easy to accept the fact that some people look down on the deaf, but it is so. They tend to equate loss of hearing with loss of reason, perhaps because of the invisibility of the handicap or a result of difficulty in communicating. It is one of the heaviest burdens deaf people have to bear.

A natural corollary to loss of hearing is loss of confidence, particularly if the person is disoriented. I therefore resolved on my return to Parliament to regain my confidence as quickly as possible. Naturally, anyone attempting this must avoid overreacting and becoming aggressive. However, provided that this danger is avoided, I regard it as of the greatest importance that deaf people should "walk tall" and not allow themselves to be patronized, however difficult the circumstances may be.

This will be easier if public attitudes toward deaf people are changed. I am aware that some deaf persons feel that it is useless to try or that it does not matter anyhow. It *does* matter, because the human environment in which deaf people live and work can eventually demoralize if it is hostile or indifferent; and it *is* worthwhile trying, because people's attitudes can and do change.

Personally, I favor anti-discrimination legislation. Although it is probably true that the law can't make people love each other, it is equally true that the law can change people's behavior. Most people are law-abiding; they discriminate unwittingly and would willingly conform to anti-discrimination legislation. I know that some anti-discrimination legislation has been enacted in the United States and other countries and that it has not been without problems. Nevertheless, such legislation constitutes an important step in the right direction and can have an important effect for the future.

Legislation will be useful, but a comprehensive change in public attitudes can only be wrought by deaf people themselves. It is by their own efforts, meeting their particular challenges, coming to terms with their unique disability, and battling to overcome their specific obstacles that deaf people can change society's view of them. People today are more enlightened about the problems of deaf people than they ever were. This is due in part to the splendid institution of Gallaudet and to the myriad voluntary organizations throughout the world. It is also due to efforts made by leaders of the deaf in all their walks of life. However, it is due primarily to deaf people themselves who are seeking to determine their own destiny.

It is the nature of the disability, and the public's perception of it, that a change in public attitudes to deafness will not be easily accomplished. But when it is achieved, the future of deaf people will be in the right hands—their own hands. They can then free themselves from patronage, discrimination, and dependency and fulfill their potentialities. That should be the aim and the aspiration of every one of us.

Chapter 5
Deafness and the Family

Pauline K. Ashley

David Wright, a deaf poet, wrote

> About deafness I know everything and nothing. Everything, if forty years'
> first-hand experience is to count. Nothing, when I realize how little I have had
> to do with the converse aspects of deafness—the other half of the dialogue. Of
> that side my wife knows more than I. (1969, p. 5)

His words make an admirable opening for any discourse on deafness; they
are particularly appropriate for one by a hearing wife.

Although I would not want to be beguiled by his eloquent prose into
accepting his argument fully, he draws welcome attention to the converse
aspect of deafness—the other half of the dialogue. Part of the deprivation
caused by deafness is inevitably experienced by the individual alone—an
obvious personal loss is that of music. But the essential significance of
deafness is that it takes away easy communication—and that is a two-way
process. If the hearing and the deaf halves of a communicating team work
together smoothly, the impact of deafness is lessened. But if the hearing half
can't or won't join in, the communication falters or fails. Conversation is
replaced by a monologue by the deaf person or, even worse, it dwindles
away, leading to greater isolation for the deaf person.

Why is it that hearing halves—members of the family and hearing
people in general—are sometimes unwilling or unable to converse with
deaf people? Why does this disability build up an impenetrable barrier?
Husbands and wives have the greatest need and motivation to communicate and, in most cases, a greater empathy. The difficulties that they face,
whether they conquer them or merely cope with them, can illuminate the
general problems of communication.

For families, total deafness is about more than communication. The
disability can affect a family in many ways, some significant and others
trivial. For the totally deaf person, however, the impact is never trivial, and
it dwarfs any possible effect on even the closest member of the family. For

the deaf person there is no respite; they have no hearing all the time. Only some of the consequences can be ameliorated, but the family can play a crucial role in this. It can provide comfort and give constant practical assistance.

When my husband lost his hearing, I believe that our close and loving family softened the blow and eased the burden of deafness. In our case, because his job was intensely oral, many practical adjustments had to be made. We tried to help in every possible way. Some were the all-important ones of assisting with lipreading; others involved knowing when to encourage him to further effort and when to suggest that he should rest and relax. It is in the subtle exercise of judgments like this that the family can be of help.

The experiences of individual members of a family involved with deafness are interrelated. Each interacts on the others, and they cannot be neatly categorized. I will first discuss some aspects of my husband's adjustment to deafness; then I will describe how his disability affected our family; and finally, I will offer a few observations on deafness in general.

SILENCE FALLS

Jack had been an MP for only 18 months when he became totally deaf following a minor ear operation. It did not occur to me or anyone else in the family that the operation might go wrong. The reduced hearing soon after the operation was worrying but readily explained by the packing in the ear canal. He coped well with an old bone-conducting hearing aid of his mother's. We were slightly worried, but we still expected the improvement in his hearing that the surgeon had confidently forecast.

A few weeks later it was Christmas, and Christmas Day was nearly normal. Using the hearing aid, Jack took the lead in the family festivities as he always did. After the worry of the previous weeks, we all relaxed and pushed aside the lurking doubts. When, on Boxing Day, his hearing collapsed, it came as a jolting shock. In the morning he had been able to talk and laugh and joke. By the afternoon he was lost in complete and fearful silence.

Together we went to the nearby ear-nose-and-throat hospital, hoping desperately for help that would transform the situation. Inevitably, as we had feared, there was no magic wand. Over many weeks the consultant tried various treatments, and we waited impatiently for an indication that one of them might work. While waiting we had to get through the interminable days with Jack existing in the eerie world of total silence.

He, of course, could talk, but there was no point in my doing so. Instead I wrote. Each day there was a pile of scribbled notes for the wastepaper basket. Books seemed tedious and irrelevant. Television and radio were out of the question. Our main diversion was the game of Scrabble. The routine of the hospital enveloped us, as it so often envelops people, but this time we seemed enclosed in a very private world of our own. The only thing that mattered was the daily hearing test.

A Scratch of Sound

The slight whisper of sound that Jack could hear taunted and tantalized as it flickered unpredictably up and down. The kind professional staff helped us as they could, but there was little that they could do and we were stressed and tested by the whole nerve-wracking business. We knew too that some harsh problems would have to be faced once we left the tranquility of the hospital. The doubts over Jack's job, and the happiness of the family, hung over us like a pall.

Fortunately, the consultant looking after him at this time, who was not the surgeon who operated, had the sense to answer our questions and respond to our fears, but not to detail the bleak implications should Jack's hearing fail to return—and I am sure now that he did not expect it to. Had we been told then what we later discovered, we would have found it difficult to cope, but we were broken in gradually to the implications and reality of deafness.

One misfortune that befell me while Jack was in hospital gave us an early warning of the nature of deafness. Leaving the hospital on a bitter cold day, I slipped on the ice and broke my wrist. It was extremely inconvenient at the time as it prevented my driving and created difficulties in my looking after our 18-month-old daughter. However, compared with near total deafness, a broken wrist is a transient and unimportant inconvenience. To our surprise, I was showered with sympathy. People probably felt—as we did—that we had enough problems already. Maybe my clearly visible injury gave others an opportunity to show the concern that they felt for Jack but which they had been unable to express.

The irony of the situation was appreciated by both of us. It demonstrated that the invisibility and the strangeness of deafness inhibits people from openly expressing sympathy. It also revealed a regrettable lack of insight and understanding about the tragedy of deafness.

Eventually it became obvious that there was not going to be any improvement in Jack's hearing. We left the hospital knowing that all medical efforts to help had failed. With the most powerful amplifier, Jack could merely hear a scratch of sound. Appallingly ill-equipped for this tragedy, he had now to face the painful adjustment to a new and unwelcome way of life.

We returned home after this traumatic experience to assess the problems waiting for us. The most urgent and dominant one was Jack's job. We both feared that his cherished Parliamentary career would have to be abandoned. Yet for Jack, Parliament was not just a job; it was a way of life that was ideal for him. From experience, he knew how ordinary people felt, and he wanted to help them from conviction and not from convenience. Jack felt at home in Parliament; his eloquence and political gifts matched the task he had set for himself. His remarkable qualifications had been universally recognized, and after only a year as an MP he had been tipped as a possible future leader of his Party. To leave Parliament would be an appalling blow. However, to stay there, Jack would have to become an outstanding lip-reader, and even that might not be good enough. There was little time to be lost; his constituency could not be without an MP much longer. Lipreading had to be learned quickly.

Learning to Lipread

Jack went to some classes, and we gathered all the books that we could find. Many were written in the last century and very few were helpful. We sought desperately for a gifted teacher but the good ones could not spare the time Jack needed. Fortunately he had a natural flair and was able to pick up a sentence from the minimum of clues. He had an almost telepathic feel of what was coming next.

His weakness was that he missed too many of the clues. To overcome this, I prepared charts for Jack that listed the various sounds in different combinations. He needed to recognize them instantaneously and this re-quired many hours of practice. We worked on it together and, as we made steady progress, our friends and neighbors helped us. It was an ad hoc, amateur approach, not entirely approved of by the professionals, but it worked.

Lipreading, if the other person was willing to help by speaking clearly, quickly became very effective. But to remain an MP, Jack had to understand all his constituents, regardless of how they spoke.

Also, at meetings, he needed a more complete tool of communication than lipreading. A good politician does not rely on words alone. Jack needed to pick up reactions, the occasional frown, the meaningful glance, the flicker of a smile and the inflection of a voice. Without these, he would find it difficult to perceive what lay beneath the words.

The common solution to a deaf person's problem of communication is to provide a signing interpreter. This would not do for Jack. An interpreter's visible presence would have struck a jarring note. More important, Jack would have had to concentrate on every sign, taking it in before it flashed into the next one. The solution we adopted—my attendance at meetings to take notes—suited us much better, and my presence was very soon taken for granted. Jack could swiftly assimilate my notes and, because the eye is faster than the voice or hand, he was left with time to look around, observe, and react to people as he had always done. The other great advantage of our system was that my place could be taken by any quick and efficient person.

However, on the other hand, there were some obvious disadvantages. Long-hand writing cannot cope with verbatim speech, and occasionally the odd misunderstanding occurred. Because the writing was done at great speed, it could be difficult to read. Fortunately, Jack's gift for making sense of scarcely perceptible lip movements stood him in good stead and he readily got the meaning of my barely comprehensible scribble.

Sometimes I found my task tiring and tedious, but more often the meetings I attended were lively and the personalities fascinating. When Jack was a member of the National Executive Committee of the Labor Party, I met the leading personalities in the Party. There were several joint meetings with the Cabinet of the then Labor Government, and I went with him to No. 10 Downing Street. Fascinated, I watched as famous politicians talked and argued with each other with all the familiarity of members of a large extended family.

Using the Phone

An essential means of communication for an MP is the telephone. Jack needed a system that could be used with any caller, required no effort from them, and ideally would work with any willing helper. The problem was resolved with a simple, extra ear piece provided by the telephone authorities. I listened to the incoming calls, repeating the words silently and simultaneously for Jack to lipread. He replied to the caller, using the normal receiver. After a little practice, the pause was only half a second or so. The system worked so well that Jack routinely does live radio interviews over the telephone.

Most people are intrigued by our telephone system, and some are baffled. They know that Jack is deaf but is apparently hearing them. "Can you hear me, Mr. Ashley?" they ask in a perplexed voice. At first, Jack would explain but now, if he is busy, he just says "Yes," and leaves them to puzzle it out. If I am not available, his secretary does the radio interviews with him—and of course she does all his business calls.

Jack is not deterred from using the phone by having no hearing person with him. He simply dials, repeatedly asks for a call back, and holds the phone while he waits. When he feels it vibrate with the ringing tone, he picks it up and gives the message. Admittedly I cannot talk to him, but a one-sided conversation is often useful.

In these various ways Jack and I worked on providing the essential tools for him to be an MP despite total deafness. He battled and adjusted to them in a remarkable way. Intensely alive to his predicament, often weary of the struggle, not only did he never give up, but he also retained his sense of fun and joy in life.

Back in Parliament

Once back in Parliament, Jack had no opportunity to take things slowly and gradually adapt to a silent world. His constituents' problems required immediate attention. A niche had to be carved out in Parliament so that fellow MPs would know that he was no lame duck. He had to keep up with politics so that his respected judgment would not falter. At the same time he needed to consolidate his lipreading, preserve his voice, and live with tinnitus. Miraculously he succeeded.

As the years passed, it became increasingly obvious that Jack was going to be a distinguished MP, not just an adequate one. He became a national figure as a result of his campaign against the company that marketed thalidomide, the drug that caused babies to be born limbless in Britain and elsewhere. The injustice being done to these children was so vividly spelled out by Jack in Parliament that the public became outraged. They organized boycotts of the firm's other products, which included a wide range of alcoholic beverages. The strength of public feeling and the loss of sales finally induced the company to pay 25 million pounds in compensation.

It was a notable victory and one that was almost as significant for Jack as for the thalidomide-damaged children. The campaign gained them the money they needed to adjust to their disability, and it showed that Jack had adjusted to his. Deafness was visibly demonstrated to be no insuperable impediment to a successful public life. In Parliament and in meetings with other campaigners, it proved to be of little consequence. Nor was it with the media. For several months, Jack's study became a press release room, and our living room a broadcasting studio.

After the thalidomide campaign, Jack became involved in many issues. Without the ties of Ministerial office he could select those that interested, moved, or outraged him. Some, such as battered wives or compensation for vaccine-damaged children, had never even been mentioned in Parliament before. In addition, he worked unstintingly for the disabled, including deaf people.

Some deaf people who have successfully secured a place in the hearing world tend to steer away from the problems of deafness, not liking to be reminded of what they have managed to avoid. But that response was not Jack's, and he fought as vigorously for deaf people as he did for others.

His achievements have been unofficially recognized by the tribute paid to him by the hundreds of people, not his constituents, who write to him every week full of confidence that he can help with their problems. On an official level, he was greatly honored by the Queen when she made him a

Companion of Honor in 1976 and a Privy Councillor in 1979. The man who 16 years ago clung on to a Parliamentary career by the thread of rudimentary lipreading is now acknowledged to be a distinguished Parliamentarian indeed.

Paradoxically, Jack may have been helped in surmounting deafness by having a job that is apparently inappropriate for a deaf person. Having chosen to stay in Parliament, where oral communication is so vital, Jack had no option but to master such communication. For him, there is no safe situation, communicating with familiar people; nearly every day he has had new people to talk to and different mouths to lipread. The pressure involved has been very great but the experience invaluable.

IMPACT ON THE FAMILY

It would be absurd to pretend that deafness has not had an impact on our family. No caring person can remain unperturbed when a close relative suffers from a profound disability. Inevitably, some of the strain we experienced when Jack first became deaf worried our two older daughters. In this sense, deafness is like any other disability, and the family had to bear with it for a while as Jack and I adjusted.

Our youngest daughter, Caroline, who was 18 months old when Jack became deaf, was virtually unaffected. The reaction of children to deafness is very refreshing. Caroline accepted it without hesitation or concern. She unceremoniously told her friends how best to speak to Jack and they calmly accepted her instruction. He loved her company and managed her childhood parties with the same energy and success that he had shown with our older daughters when he had had his hearing.

We were fortunate in that deafness did not cause a change of job, as it undoubtedly does in many circumstances. Deaf people who suffer both loss of hearing and loss of job must be in a desperate plight, and their families must suffer with them both emotionally and in practical ways.

The major concern of our family has been to ensure easy communication with Jack. We all wanted him to remain closely involved in family life, aware of the trivial as well as the important events.

At first it wasn't easy. As with his constituency meetings, we wondered about having sign language to use within the family. It would have ensured complete communication and once we had become adept, no doubt we would all have found it easier and more relaxing. However, we knew that in the outside world, especially in Parliament, lipreading, despite its weaknesses, had to be his main form of communication; therefore, it had to be so within the family. In the early days, Jack insisted that we should speak normally so that there would be no contrast with other people. We found it difficult to resist an instinctive desire to make lipreading easier by mouthing. His repeated phrase, "Don't mouth," was irritating to all of us, but he was right to press his point. Once the lipreading was well established we all relaxed a little, no longer feeling that home conversation was essential lipreading practice.

To us, our family conversation appears virtually normal. It is routine to make sure that Jack is looking before we speak. As names are difficult to lipread, we preface one by indicating that it is a name. If necessary, we spell it quickly—one way or another. This keeps the momentum of the conversation going. We learned by experience that a stop-go conversation could all too easily become a stopped one!

Fatigue

One of our few unsolved problems has been the effect of fatigue, which deafness so easily brings, especially when it is accompanied by tinnitus and when life is full of pressures requiring instant responses. When Jack is tired, inevitably his lipreading skill declines, and the extra effort required adds to his exhaustion. This spiral places the family in a quandary. We hesitate over whether something is worth saying or not. Does it justify the lipreading effort involved? The alternative is silence; would that be better, or would it be depressing and perhaps misunderstood? There are no easy answers. We find we can only use our judgment. Sometimes we get it right and sometimes not.

Similar problems can occur if we are rushed. When the doorbell rings and the telephone goes and there is a smell of burning from the kitchen, it hardly seems sensible to stop and explain the detail of what is happening to Jack. Fortunately his perceptions are so quick that the conflicting needs rarely produce a real dilemma.

Leisure activities lead to difficulties of a different kind. With memories of the long tedious days in hospital, I was apprehensive at first about how we would spend our spare time. It was an unnecessary concern.

Most leisure activities involve physical exertion, on which Jack thrives, or social chat. To my delight, I find that our friends enjoy our company as much as they ever did. Sometimes they enjoy it too much! Regrettably, it is my eyes that droop, while Jack, who has to bear the strain of lipreading, talks on late into the night with our happily oblivious friends.

There is no real difficulty for our family in relaxing and watching television just as so many other families do. In Britain, many programs now have subtitles, and for those we want to watch that have none, the additional note is no hardship. Sometimes, though, we may balance the pleasure long programs will give against the effort of notetaking. Sport on television requires no subtitles or notes, and Jack is a great television sports fan.

In the early stressful years of deafness, watching Saturday afternoon sports was Jack's main relaxation. He enjoyed watching horse racing and often put the British equivalent of a couple of dollars on his selections. I would listen to the commentary and help him follow the race on our black and white set. Unfortunately, I see horses as identical four-legged animals, which made me a hopeless race reader. Consequently Jack often missed the pleasure of watching his horse win, because I had indicated that it was at the back of the field rather than up with the leaders. To my relief, we bought a color television. With that he could follow the horses himself and my contribution was reduced to rejoicing when he won and—more often—commiserating when he lost!

The handful of tedious problems that have arisen for the family have been due to the combination of deafness and politics. For example, our telephone is always ringing. I have often been waked at 6 in the morning by apologetic but determined journalists seeking a story before their early deadline. They wake me, and then I have to decide whether or not to wake Jack, a weary husband who may only have got to bed a few hours earlier.

Personally, I find the flood of calls that accompany a lively political campaign more troublesome. Each requires some help for Jack. On those days the household chores are forgotten.

Deafness has altered my domestic role in other ways. When I accompanied Jack to his constituency in the years when the children were young, my mother and sister took over the household responsibilities; my mother would stay during the day and my working sister for the night. We were fortunate that they were able to help us in this way. It enabled us to concentrate on the constituency work, knowing that the children were not suffering from our absence.

Effects on the Hearing

Although the effects of deafness on the family are interesting and important, they have not really been explored. Among the views I have encountered, a remarkable one comes from David Wright, whom I mentioned earlier. He says that " . . . it is the nondeaf who absorb a large part of the impact of the disability." It is a plausible theory. Conversation is an interdependent and responsive thing, and, when one person is deaf, it can be demanding on the other.

However, all disabilities, by their nature, are stressful. There is nothing to suggest that deafness is uniquely more difficult for the spouse than for the sufferer. In my view, it is absurd to compare, as Wright does, the minor inconvenience experienced by one with the profound deprivation suffered by the other.

Since the views of deaf people themselves are so conflicting, it is not surprising that hearing people have a confusing picture of the implications of total deafness. It appears to most people to be a strange and baffling complaint that should be avoided if possible.

Even Jack, an exceptional person who is so well established in the hearing world, meets this reaction quite regularly. I noticed that when he first became deaf and his lipreading was still a little primitive, someone needing his help or advice would always manage to communicate. But when it came to general conversation, the same person would suddenly find communication more difficult.

There is an instinctive tendency for hearing people to turn and talk to those who can hear rather than to those who cannot, even when the conversation concerns the deaf person. However good or bad the lipreading skill of the deaf person, deafness creates a social barrier that has to be demolished. Sometimes the hearing person will do it with no difficulty; more often it is left to the one who is deaf. This is not always an easy task, for it requires a delicate touch, humor, and confidence, but it must be devoid of brashness.

Sometimes another person can help. When I accompany Jack, I do what I can to reduce the difficulties, but my presence can be counterproductive. Many people are intrigued to meet him because he is a well-known public figure. They greet him with enthusiasm, but at the first lipreading difficulty, they turn to me and say, "Tell him what I said. He follows you better." That may be true, but it is an unsatisfactory way to converse.

My tactics for dealing with this vary with the individual. I usually start by keeping my eyes on Jack's face as they talk to me. Disconcerted, they switch their gaze and start talking to him. If that doesn't work, I politely say directly, "If you talk to Jack, it's easier for him to lipread." With gentle reminders if they slip back into talking through me, we usually manage to get a "proper" conversation, satisfying to both sides and with deafness in its proper place—an inconvenience rather than a barrier.

Sometimes I am less successful in helping Jack. On social occasions I may be acting as both a participant and an interpreter. It is only too easy to fulfill just one of the roles. I am rather a single-minded person and, if I get absorbed in conversation, tend to become oblivious of what is going on around me. Fortunately, I have learned to participate in one conversation while simultaneously being aware of another. In this way I can help Jack quickly should it be necessary.

If a deaf person is to be assisted, it needs to be done with consideration of their sensibilities. Nothing is worse than the "aren't I being good" pose. Some people are willing to help but they want everyone to know it and they behave ostentatiously. One or two MPs have been quoted in the press as saying how helpful their signals to Jack had been in Parliament. These claims were made by those who were least helpful. On the other hand, MPs who took a great deal of trouble never sought credit for it.

Reactions to deafness can be perplexing. I have known people who, after being with Jack for an hour or so, comment that he doesn't seem to be a deaf person. This is despite an occasional, or even frequent, hiccup with lipreading. They are paying him a compliment, but the implication is no compliment to deaf people in general. What they have noticed is that Jack does not feel inferior because of deafness, and therefore he never behaves in the slightly humbled way that the struggle to understand so often induces in the deaf person. With a temperament that is a mix of aggression, warmth, and humor, he is constitutionally incapable of allowing others to dominate him.

SELF-CONFIDENCE

Self-confidence is perhaps the key to the management of deafness, and Jack is fortunate in having an abundance of it. Who else would go into an unknown flower shop, as he once did, and say, "I want to send my wife a bouquet of flowers, and I've come out without my checkbook. Will you trust me?" Most hearing people would hesitate, to say nothing of deaf people who are uncertain about lipreading the reply. But Jack is always willing to have a go, and his confidence is usually repaid, as it was in this case.

I suspect that few totally deaf people have as much self-confidence as Jack, for confidence is a frail thing, laboriously established and easily whittled away. The situation is further complicated by its chicken and egg relationship with deafness. A diffident person, slightly apologetic about being deaf, tends to provoke irritation, causing him or her a further loss of confidence. In contrast, a relaxed person, briskly treating deafness as a problem to be overcome, generates a constructive response, thus boosting his or her confidence.

The popular image of deafness is no help to the deaf. Many advertisements for hearing aids portray deafness as a disability to be ashamed of, one that should be tucked away. The so-called invisibility of deafness sometimes deludes deaf people into thinking that they can hide it. Some can, although I doubt if they gain much by it. Generally, with uncompensated deafness, the bluff is only too apparent to hearing people, and the only one deluded is the deaf person. But perhaps this is an area in which only the deaf understand the problem, and the desire to make deafness invisible is a necessary defensive reaction to the behavior of hearing people.

The real issue with deafness is not whether or not it can be concealed but how its consequences can be minimized. This requires a greater knowledge and understanding of deafness, and a modification of the attitudes of both the deaf and the hearing.

Jack's presence in Parliament has helped deaf people in Britain in various ways. Because total deafness is rare, there is a tendency among some hearing people not familiar with it to equate total deafness with abnormality. Jack's many appearances on radio and television have had the beneficial effect of demonstrating to millions that a totally deaf person is still a normal human being who can laugh and joke and protest and argue with the best of them.

Some deaf people have been encouraged by his public role; I am sure that, for at least a few, he has raised their expectations of what life can hold. Although his example is unlikely to be followed until technical progress in translating the spoken word has made the task easier, he has shown that even the improbable is possible.

Deaf people are of course as varied in their talents and their temperaments as hearing people. Their expectations, and those of their families for them, should stretch but not break them—and that requires a perceptive understanding of both the individual talent and the constraints of deafness. If these are realistically assessed by deaf people and their families, they will be well equipped to face this crippling disability. Deaf people can then simultaneously use their talents to the full and come to terms with deafness.

REFERENCE

Wright, D. (1969). *Deafness* (p. 5). New York: Stein and Day.

PART III

ADJUSTMENT TO HEARING LOSS

Chapter **6**
Benefits and Limitations of Amplification and Speechreading for the Elderly

Harriet Kaplan

Hearing loss is widespread among the elderly. In the United States, approximately 55 per cent of adults with hearing loss severe enough to interfere with receptive communication are age 65 or over (Berkowitz, 1975). Maurer and Rupp (1979) state, "One of every two members of the large retiree population has a hearing problem that is interfering with communicative ability and lifestyle goals, and four out of five . . . are experiencing some communicative problems in listening."

The majority have sensorineural hearing loss, which is not amenable to medical or surgical treatment. Many younger adults with such a loss benefit greatly from amplification and associated aural rehabilitation. Similar benefits might be expected for the elderly, but hearing aids are not usually as successful with this group. In 1950 Carhart called the geriatric population a "problem population." Let us consider why this is so and what can be done about it.

To be used optimally, amplification should be part of a comprehensive aural rehabilitation program. This is true for all adults, but particularly the elderly. Therefore, I will first discuss issues involved in the successful use of amplification and factors that may indicate if an individual is a good hearing aid candidate. I will then discuss other aspects of rehabilitation, including assistive devices, hearing aid orientation, communication strategies, speechreading or lipreading, manipulating the listening environment, and the involvement of family and friends.

FACTORS AFFECTING SUCCESSFUL HEARING AID USE

It is important to realize the tremendous variability among people over 65 years of age, in lifestyle, degree of hearing loss and handicap, communicative needs, personality, physical and mental problems—and, of course, age. All these factors affect the use of amplification. Therefore, each individual must be evaluated and appropriate recommendations made, based on his or her distinctive condition.

Rupp, Higgins, and Maurer (1977) have developed a "Feasibility Scale for Predicting Hearing Aid Use" involving evaluation of many prognostic factors. They consider motivation the single most important factor. Does the individual truly want help? Does he consider his hearing loss a handicap? Who is really experiencing the problem, the hearing-impaired person or family members who cannot easily communicate with him? The authors point out that persons who really want help are more likely to use a hearing aid successfully than those urged on by others. The elderly patient who tells the audiologist, "My daughter thinks I need a hearing aid," may not be ready to use one.

Motivation is related to lifestyle. The person who is active physically, mentally, and emotionally and participates in community affairs, and who perhaps retains some employment, needs to communicate and will have a strong desire to adjust to amplification. The withdrawn person who spends most of his time alone usually will not—unless he depends on the telephone and television.

Elderly persons often minimize the handicap of hearing loss or project its problems onto others: "I can hear if you would talk clearly." Maurer and Rupp (1979) feel that the more realistic the individual's self-assessment is, the better the prognosis for remediation. A number of scales for the self-assessment of communication difficulties are available (Alpiner, Chevrette, Glascoe, Metz, and Olsen, 1975; Giolas, Owens, Lamb, and Schubert, 1982; High, Fairbanks, and Glorig, 1964; Noble and Atherly, 1970; Noble, 1978; Ventry and Weinstein, 1982). If the subjective perception of the effects of hearing loss matches objective predictions based on audiometric data, the prognosis for successful hearing aid use is improved.

Assessment scales indicate the situations that pose communication problems and the individual's attitudes toward them. A scale should be used early in therapy to clarify the prognosis for amplification and focus the aural rehabilitation program. It identifies desirable modifications in the listening environment, aids in deciding whether an assistive device may be preferable to a hearing aid, and helps to guide speechreading training, communication strategies, and the counseling of relatives and friends.

Many people do not clearly understand what a hearing aid can and cannot do. They expect it to restore normal hearing, but no aid can do so for a person with a sensorineural hearing loss. There are two types of hearing problems: one of loudness and one of clarity. Amplification can deal only with the former. In the latter type of hearing problem, speech at normal or near-normal levels is heard but not clearly understood, because it is distorted. The vast majority of hearing-impaired adults, both young and old, experience both problems. By increasing the volume or intensity of speech, amplification can improve sound reception but it does not eliminate distortion. Speech understanding is improved but not restored to normal. Unless this limitation is accepted, the person will be disappointed with, and may not use, the hearing aid. An evaluation of the ability to discriminate or understand comfortably loud speech is an important part of a thorough audiological examination.

Amplification may improve speechreading and, for the profoundly impaired, restore coupling to the world of sound; this is important to those who have had normal hearing for most of their life. Recognizing environmental sounds such as the sound of a door closing or a car horn increases the individual's sense of security.

In summary, before a hearing aid is bought, an audiological examination should define the benefits and limitations of amplification and the situations in which it can be used successfully.

A hearing aid does not function well in a noisy setting; it picks up and amplifies any sound within its range. In such a setting, a user must sort out the amplified speech from the amplified noise. Hearing persons do so, to some degree, with two ears; with the "built-in distortion" of damaged hearing, and using only one hearing aid, it is far more difficult. Binaural amplification often helps, but cannot resolve, the problem of speech discrimination in noise.

Because of the limitations of amplification, a hearing aid user must adapt to the different sound it provides, manipulate the controls, insert the earmold and battery, take care of the instrument, and perform simple troubleshooting. Elderly people, particularly the institutionalized elderly, tend to show reduced flexibility and adaptability. The more adaptable an individual is, the better the prognosis for successful use of amplification.

Use of a hearing aid requires a certain manual dexterity, which may decline with age. Three general problems can interfere with hearing aid management by the elderly:

1. Reduced tactile sensitivity hampers the manipulation of very small controls and the secure insertion of the earmold.

2. Reduced mobility of fingers, hands, and arms, often caused by arthritis, hampers adjusting the volume control, battery compartment, or telephone switch.

3. Slower neuromuscular responses may make it impossible to turn down the volume control quickly upon sudden exposure to loud noise (Maurer and Rupp, 1979). These problems can deter successful use of amplification, particularly in a nursing home.

A dependable spouse, child, friend, or aide can assume much responsibility for managing the hearing aid, or an aid can be selected with large, accessible controls. However, most people want a small and inconspicuous hearing aid. Elderly persons rarely accept a body-type aid with controls that are easy to manipulate. Even a behind-the-ear aid may be rejected for an in-the-ear type.

Another reason for resistance to a hearing aid is its perceived social stigma. Even an inconspicuous aid can signify "growing old," which is not valued in our society. Hence, whatever the communicative penalty, the elderly person may try to deny his or her hearing loss. Wax (1982) discusses the "double jeopardy" of the elderly, who experience the inter-acting effects of two devalued statuses, age and deafness.

The lack of success with many hearing aids is attributable to their purchase from unscrupulous dispensers without advice from a physician or audiologist. Isolated elderly persons are often victimized in this manner. In some cases, professionals do not take the time to adequately evaluate and counsel the elderly with hearing problems.

Even mild or moderate presbycusis, the hearing loss due to aging, may severely reduce speech discrimination ability. This phenomenon of pho-nemic regression was first identified in 1948 by John Gaeth and later substantiated by Pestalozza and Shore (1955) and Goetzinger, Proud, Dirks, and Embry (1961). Although more recent research has not identi-fied phonemic regression in the majority of the elderly hearing-impaired, it can be a serious problem in individual cases (Bergman, 1971; Harbert, Young, and Menduke, 1966; Kasden, 1970).

Far more prevalent are effects of aging on the perception of degraded speech. In the presence of noise or other conditions interfering with optimal transmission, the speech discrimination of elderly hearing-impaired persons deteriorates dramatically. In comprehensive studies, Bergman (1980) manipulated physical aspects of the message to provide different degrees of signal degradation. Interrupting speech, slowing it down, speeding it up, removing high frequencies, masking speech with noise or babble, and creating reverberation, he found a disproportionally greater problem in elderly than in younger adults with the same level of hearing loss. A monaural hearing aid limited understanding in both groups, especially the elderly. Jerger (1973) found that presbycusic subjects un-derstood faint speech, time-compressed speech, and speech presented against a competing message less well than younger adults with the same decibel loss. Antonelli (1970), Blumenfeld, Bergman, and Millner (1969), Orchik and Burgess (1977), Kirikae (1969), and Smith and Prather (1971) report similar results.

The implications are clear. The limitations of amplification systems are complicated by the nature of hearing loss in the elderly. Elderly persons vary in their ability to discriminate speech in quiet and against competing signals. Presbycusis is not a single entity. In postmortem temporal bone studies, Schuknecht (1955, 1964) identified four distinct pathological processes, three in sites in the inner ear and one in the central auditory pathways of the brain. The degree and configuration of pure tone hearing loss and discrimination ability differed in each type. Others have supported these findings; excellent discussions can be found in Maurer and Rupp (1979, Chapter 3) and Beasley and Davis (1981, Chapters 14 and 15).

The person with severe discrimination problems in noise may nevertheless benefit from a hearing aid in situations involving one-to-one communication, watching television, and using the telephone.

Many factors governing successful hearing aid use apply to younger as well as older adults. However, the former are less likely to deny their hearing loss or withdraw into isolation; since it is necessary for them to communicate at work, they are more likely to seek help; also, they are more likely to be adaptable and dexterous, and their loss (except when noise-induced) does not usually pose severe discrimination-in-noise problems. Hence, they usually respond better to amplification.

Many limitations of amplification can be overcome by a comprehensive aural rehabilitation program, which will be outlined in the remainder of this chapter.

HEARING AID ORIENTATION

Hearing aid orientation provides the information and counseling needed to use an aid properly. First and foremost, it includes information about what the aid can reasonably be expected to do, which will vary with the individual's hearing loss. Someone with good unaided speech discrimination in both quiet and noise will gain significantly improved understanding in most situations. The individual with poor unaided discrimination will improve less in speech understanding, but may still function better, particularly if he also uses speechreading and communication strategies. A person with good discrimination in quiet but not in noise may use a hearing aid successfully on a part-time basis. Each must be helped to appreciate his or her own condition.

Counseling should start before a hearing aid is fitted and continue throughout the hearing aid evaluation and adjustment period, however long it may last. The audiologist should help the individual with any problems that arise with a new aid. A program of carefully guided listening activities may sometimes be employed so that easy listening will precede more difficult situations. Group therapy and support groups provide useful peer support.

During the adjustment period, modifications of hearing aid settings may be necessary. The internal adjustment of an aid or an earmold can help to alleviate a noise problem or a feeling of discomfort. The need for such modifications will become apparent as the aid is used in everyday situations.

Training is necessary in the use and care of the hearing aid. Often, after only one session an elderly person does not use the controls or insert the battery or earmold properly. Instructions must be repeated and the individual given hands-on practice under supervision. A family member may help the hearing aid user to master the instrument.

For all these reasons, the elderly person needs ongoing contact with the audiologist to ensure successful hearing aid use. Lack of such contact is one reason why so many aids end up in dresser drawers.

ASSISTIVE DEVICES

In noisy or reverberant rooms, hearing aids provide minimal to moderate benefits. In a typical meeting room, lecture hall, church, or theater, speech can reach the ear or the hearing aid microphone at only a slightly louder level than background noise. A public address system will raise the loudness or intensity but will introduce distortions. For an elderly person who has difficulty understanding speech against background noise, these conditions can present an intolerable situation. A hearing aid, which may serve well in a quiet environment, is of little value. The individual with a hearing loss too mild to warrant use of amplification can also have trouble discerning speech against background noise. Similar problems occur for many hearing-impaired people listening to transmitting equipment of variable fidelity, such as the telephone, radio, or television, and to voices in competing noise or reverberation.

These problems can be resolved by improving the signal-to-noise ratio, enabling the speech to reach the ear at a significantly louder level than the noise, as undistorted as possible. This is precisely what an assistive device does. Such a device is any system, aside from a hearing aid, that improves the communication of the hearing-impaired. A high-fidelity microphone close to a speaker will pick up his speech better than background noise. The speech signal is then amplified and delivered to the ear by direct wire, magnetic inductive pickup (the telephone circuit of a hearing aid used with a loop), FM transmission, or infrared transmission, which is similar to FM but uses light waves instead of radio frequencies. The listener picks up the signal with a hearing aid or earphones connected to the device.

Assistive devices may be designed for the following:

1. Large groups. Devices such as an induction loop used with the telephone circuit of a hearing aid, FM systems similar to auditory trainers

used by deaf children in some schools, and infrared transmission can be connected to existing public address systems.

2. Personal listening in noise, usually utilizing FM transmission or hardwire connection between a microphone and the amplifier, receiver, or earphone unit. Again, the key factor is the microphone close to the speaker. A number of situations can be handled well with these devices. Many senior citizens eat in communal areas such as cafeterias or dining halls, where the clatter of dishes and babble of talk render a hearing aid useless; however, the assistive device with an external microphone makes conversation possible. In an automobile, conversation is affected by noise and also by the fact that the driver cannot face the listener; an external microphone is an excellent solution. The difficulty of conversing around a conference table or out-of-doors can be overcome in the same way.

3. Telephone listening. Relief from a signal of low volume and fidelity and background noise can be obtained by built-in or portable amplifiers, use of the hearing aid induction coil, eliminating room noise, or various teletype devices.

4. Using the television or radio. Placing a microphone at the sound source or, better, connecting the television or radio to the amplifier or receiver of the assistive device minimizes room noise and allows the listener to adjust the volume on his amplifier or aid. Thus, he or she can listen at one volume while family members listen at another and all can be comfortable. Hardwire, loops, infrared, or FM may be used. A special device brings closed captioning to the TV screen.

5. Signaling the telephone, doorbell, alarm clock, smoke alarm, baby's crib, and so forth, by flashing light, extremely loud sound (e.g., a gong), or vibration. A microphone picks up the monitored sound by inductive sensing or a hardwire connection and can deliver it to an immediate or remote receiver.

Assistive devices can substitute for or supplement hearing aids in situations where aids alone are of little value. An excellent discussion of these devices can be found in Vaughn, Lightfoot, and Gibbs (1983).

MANIPULATING THE LISTENING ENVIRONMENT

Sometimes, modifying the listening environment can ease communication. For example, the TV volume should be turned down before answering the phone. To improve or avoid other situations, such as talking to someone in one room while the water is running or while others are talking in another, the understanding and cooperation of family and friends may be needed.

Good room acoustics can help. Drapes, carpets, and soundproofed walls and ceilings that reduce reverberation that interferes with speech clarity are particularly important in communal areas of nursing homes, senior citizen centers, clubs, and other gathering places.

INVOLVEMENT OF FAMILY AND FRIENDS

Family and friends can play a critical part in the rehabilitation process if they understand the effects of noise, acoustics, poor lighting and mumbled speech on communication with the hearing-impaired, and why a deafened person can hear some things easily but not others. Therefore, audiologists commonly encourage a spouse, child, or other relative or a friend to enter the rehabilitation program with their client; indeed, Hardick (1977) will not accept an unaccompanied client in his program. Most participants in the Gallaudet Elderhostel program are accompanied by a spouse or friend. Hull (1982) encourages family members to be fitted with ear plugs to understand hearing loss better.

By identifying home situations that create special hearing difficulties, family members can act together to minimize them without disrupting the life of the household. By understanding the limitations of amplification and the time needed to adjust to it, the family can provide vital help in a troubling period.

In a nursing home, the in-service training of aides, volunteers, and nurses should focus on the use and care of hearing aids and earmolds and how to communicate with hearing-impaired residents. Much hands-on practice is important to effective training.

SPEECHREADING OR LIPREADING

In 1930 Nitchie defined speechreading as "the art of understanding a speaker's thoughts by watching the movements of his mouth"; subsequent studies have shown that facial expressions are equally significant (Greenberg and Bode, 1968; Stone, 1957). Speechreading is a synthetic, cognitive skill which integrates visible facial movements with other available information to grasp the speaker's words and thoughts. It exploits the characteristics and the redundancies of the language and the situation, including the following:

1. What is audible. Most hard-of-hearing adults can hear many speech sounds. For example, p, b, and m are difficult to discriminate visually but not aurally and people with moderate hearing loss can often distinguish them. Similarly, vowel differences are difficult to see but easy to hear. Several studies have shown that speech with visual cues is perhaps 20 per cent more intelligible than speech alone (Binnie, 1973, 1974; Erber, 1969,

1972). Speechreading is not a substitute for, but an adjunct to, amplification (see Berger, 1978; Binnie, 1976; Jeffers and Barley, 1971; O'Neill and Oyer, 1981, Chapter 7).

2. Gestures, facial expressions, and body language. The few pertinent studies indicate a significant increase in understanding with appropriate bodily clues (Berger and Popelka, 1971; Popelka and Berger, 1971).

3. Situational or contextual clues. Information about the setting, role, and status of speakers helps participants to anticipate and interpret what is said.

4. Language structure. In any sentence, some words fit linguistically, while others do not. The rules governing word order, syntactic forms such as negation, and possible combinations of phonemes facilitate speechreading.

The good speechreader cannot rely exclusively on visible phoneme movements, because poor lighting, distance, and obstructions may interfere with his view of the speaker. Under common viewing conditions, about 60 per cent of speech sounds are obscure or invisible (Jeffers and Barley, 1971); many words—such as mat, bat, pat—look alike; normal speech is rapid and blurs movements that may be visible with slower speech. Therefore, successful speechreading requires the ability to synthesize varied cues rapidly, which is primarily a cognitive talent.

People vary in their ability to use communication redundancies. Garstecki (1979) found that some elderly people ignore, misinterpret, or are distracted by situational cues and require training to use them in everyday situations. Cooper (1979) noted that many are reluctant to watch a speaker's face.

There seems to be a negative relationship between speechreading and age. Simmons (1959) compared age and speechreading skill in a group of hard-of-hearing adults with a mean age of 47; older subjects tended to be poorer speechreaders, although the correlation was not statistically significant. Goetzinger (1963) also found age and speechreading to be negatively associated; his older subjects were poorer speechreaders.

Other studies have indicated that visual perception declines with age. Speechreading ability tends to decline with age, especially beyond middle age (Ewertson and Nielsen, 1971; Farrimond, 1959); it is not clear whether physiological or psychological factors or both are responsible. Schuknecht (1964) demonstrated that general neural atrophy underlies the decline in auditory speech processing ability; a similar atrophy may affect the visual system. Farrimond attributed speechreading decline to changes in the central nervous processes due to aging. Some studies suggest that speechreading deteriorates as visual acuity deteriorates (Lovering and Hardick, 1969; Hardick, Oyer, and Irion, 1970) due to presbyopia, cataracts, retinal disorders, and glaucoma. Others report decreased speechreading ability with age even though visual acuity is held constant (Ewertsen and Nielsen, 1971; Farrimond, 1959; Pelson and Prather, 1974). Pelson and Prather showed that the visual perception of spoken sentences, when the speaker was seen but not heard, was better among younger hearing persons than among older hearing or hearing-impaired persons.

Shoop and Binnie (1978) evaluated the sentence speechreading ability of 110 normal-hearing adults divided into four older groups (40 to 50, 51 to 60, 61 to 70, and over 70 years of age) and a younger group (20 to 23 years old). The younger group was significantly best in the visual perception of sentences; the ability of the four older groups deteriorated with age; those ages 40 to 50 and 51 to 60 performed similarly, but those 61 to 70 years of age were significantly poorer, and the oldest group, over age 70, was poorer still.

Schow, Christensen, Hutchinson, and Nerbonne (1978) summarized several experiments documenting the visual processing difficulties of the elderly. These difficulties may arise because of peripheral changes—the central nervous system receiving less information for its processing decisions—or because changes in the central nervous system reduce its ability to integrate information from one or several senses. Older people may respond slowly and rigidly, with a reduced ability to change percepts, whereas rapid responses and flexible speech percepts are necessary for good speechreading. In addition, experiments suggest that older subjects require much greater exposure time to identify designs, words, or pictures (Riegel, 1956; Wallace, 1956).

Although proficiency deteriorates with age, older persons can still benefit from speechreading. The necessary training should focus on practical, real-life situations, and attentiveness to a speaker's face and situational and communicative redundancies. The individual should know the possibilities and limitations of speechreading and learn how to improve communication by manipulating the environment.

COMMUNICATION STRATEGIES

Communication strategies include all methods of coping with difficult situations: planning ahead, manipulating the environment, and various repair techniques.

Planning ahead involves anticipating and trying to minimize difficulties. For example, an individual planning to attend a lecture may familiarize himself with the topic, ask the speaker to use the microphone and keep his face visible, and arrive early to get a good seat. As another example, an individual taking a car to the garage may try to anticipate the terms the mechanic will use and ask a friend to say them aloud.

Manipulating the environment includes steps such as asking a speaker to move into the light or to a quieter spot, turning off the television or radio during conversation, moving closer to a speaker or asking him to remove gum or a cigarette from his mouth.

Repair techniques include obtaining important information in writing; asking a speaker to repeat or rephrase a remark or spell a word or number; and asking him or her, "Did you say . . . ?"

To employ these techniques, a person must be assertive, admit a hearing problem, and specify the actions required. Many elderly people grow passive, particularly in a nursing home, and need help to become more assertive. Group programs where participants support each other are a good way to accomplish this.

Sources that discuss the foregoing strategies include Bower and Bower (1976), Harrelson (1982), Hull (1982), Jacobs (1979), Kaplan (1982a,b), McCarthy and Alpiner (1978), and Rupp and Heavenrich (1982).

CONCLUSION

Successful use of amplification by elderly persons is affected by the nature of presbycusis, other disabilities, the individual's lifestyle, and his perceptions of hearing loss and aging. All elderly persons are not good hearing aid candidates. Often, motivation to use amplification can be developed by participation in a group program. Amplification should be viewed as part of a comprehensive aural rehabilitation program, which will vary from individual to individual.

The first step in such a program is assessment of the hearing loss, the individual's attitudes toward himself, and his specific communication problems. A program to remediate these problems can then be developed, including, as needed, hearing and orientation, family involvement, environmental manipulation, speechreading, communication strategies, and assistive devices. If rehabilitation is approached broadly and with attention to each individual's special needs and circumstances, rather than as merely hearing aid fitting, most elderly persons can be at least partially helped to overcome the deleterious effects of hearing loss.

REFERENCES

Alpiner, J., Chevrette, W., Glascoe, G., Metz, M., and Olsen, B. (1975). The Denver Scale of Communication Function. In M. Pollack (Ed.), *Amplification for the hearing impaired* (pp. 176-183). New York: Grune and Stratton.

Antonelli, A. R. (1970). Sensitized speech tests in aged people. In C. Rojskjaer (Ed.), *Speech audiometry* (pp. 66-79). Second Danavox Symposium, Odense, Denmark.

Beasley, D. S., and Davis, G. A. (1981). *Aging: Communication processes and disorders.* New York: Grune and Stratton.

Berger, K. W. (1978). Speechreading, principles and methods (Ch. 3-4). Kent, OH: Herald Publisher.

Berger, K. W., and Popelka, G. R. (1971). Extra-facial gestures in relation to speechreading. *Journal of Communication Disorders, 3,* 302-308.

Bergman, M. (1971). Hearing and aging, *Audiology, 10,* 164-171.

Bergman, M. (1980) *Aging and perception of speech.* Baltimore: University Park Press.

Berkowitz, A. (1975). Audiological rehabilitation of the geriatric patient. *Hearing Aid Journal, 8,* 30-34.

Binnie, C. A. (1973). Bisensory articulation functions for normal hearing and sensorineural hearing loss patients. *Journal of the Academy of Rehabilitative Audiology, 6,* 43-53.

Binnie, C. A. (1974). Auditory-visual intelligibility of various speech materials presented in three noise backgrounds. In H. B. Nielsen and E. Kampp (Eds.), *Visual and audio-visual perception of speech. Scandinavian Audiology* (Suppl. 4), 255-280.

Binnie, C. A. (1976). Relevant aural rehabilitation. In J. L. Northern (Ed.), *Hearing disorders* (Ch. 20). Boston: Little, Brown.

Blumenfeld, V. G., Bergman, M., and Millner, E. (1969). Speech discrimination in an aging population. *Journal of Speech and Hearing Research, 12,* 210-217.

Bower, S. A., and Bower, G. H. (1976). *Asserting yourself: A practical guide for positive change.* Reading, MA: Addison-Wesley.

Carhart, R. (1950). Hearing aid selection by university clinics. *Journal of Speech and Hearing Disorders, 15,* 105-113.

Cooper, J. C. (1979). Aural rehabilitation: Philosophy, rationale, and technique. In M. Henoch (Ed.), *Aural rehabilitation for the elderly* (pp. 31-52). New York: Grune and Stratton.

Erber, N. P. (1969). Interaction of audition and vision in the recognition of speech material. *Journal of Speech and Hearing Research, 12,* 423-425.

Erber, N. P. (1972). Auditory, visual and auditory-visual recognition of consonants by children with normal and impaired hearing. *Journal of Speech and Hearing Research, 17,* 413-422.

Ewertsen, H. W., and Nielsen, H. B. (1971). A comparative analysis of the audiovisual, auditive and visual perception of speech. *Acta Otolaryngologica, 72,* 201-205.

Farrimond, T. (1959). Age differences in the ability to use visual cues in auditory communication. *Language and Speech, 2,* 179-192.

Gaeth, J. (1948). *A study of phonemic regression in relation to hearing loss.* Unpublished doctoral dissertation, Northwestern University, Evanston, IL.

Garstecki, D. C. (1979). The use of situational cues in visual communication. In M. Henoch (Ed.), *Aural rehabilitation for the elderly* (pp. 31-52). New York: Grune and Stratton.

Giolas, T., Owens, E., Lamb, S. H., and Schubert, E. (1982). Hearing performance inventory. In T. G. Giolas (Ed.), *Hearing handicapped adults* (pp. 189-199). Englewood Cliffs, NJ: Prentice-Hall.

Goetzinger, C. P. (1963). A study of monocular versus binocular vision in lipreading. *Proceedings of the International Congress on Education of the Deaf and 41st Meeting of the Convention of American Instructors of the Deaf* (pp. 326-333). Washington, DC: U.S. Government Printing Office.

Goetzinger, C. P., Proud, G. O., Dirks, D., and Embry, J. (1961). A study of hearing in advanced age. *AMA Archives of Otolaryngology, 73,* 662-674.

Greenberg, J. J., and Bode, D. L. (1968). Visual discrimination of consonants. *Journal of Speech and Hearing Research, 11,* 869-874.

Harbert, R., Young, I., and Menduke, H. (1966). Audiological findings in presbycusis. *Journal of Auditory Research, 9,* 159-166.

Hardick, E. (1977). Aural rehabilitation programs for the aged can be successful. *Journal of the Academy of Rehabilitative Audiology, 10,* 51-66.

Hardick, E. J., Oyer, H. J., and Irion, P. E. (1970). Lipreading performance as related to measurement of vision. *Journal of Speech and Hearing Research, 13,* 92-100.

Harrelson, L. M. (1982, October). Strategies for the hearing impaired. *Hearing Instruments, 33,* 9-10.

High, W. S., Fairbanks, G., and Glorig, A. (1964). Scale for self-assessment of hearing handicap. *Journal of Speech and Hearing Disorders, 29,* 215-230.

Hull, R. H. (1982). Techniques of aural rehabilitation treatment for elderly clients. In R. H. Hull (Ed.), *Rehabilitative audiology* (pp. 383-406). New York: Grune and Stratton.

Jacobs, M. (1979). *Speechreading strategies.* Rochester, NY: National Technical Institute for the Deaf.

Jeffers, J., and Barley, M. (1971). *Speechreading (lipreading)* (pp. 150-186). Springfield, IL: Charles C Thomas.

Jerger, J. (1973). Audiological findings in aging. *Advances in Oto-Rhino-Laryngology, 20,* 115-124.

Kaplan, H. (1982a). Facilitating adjustment. In R. H. Hull (Ed.), *Rehabilitative audiology* (pp. 81-97). New York: Grune and Stratton.

Kaplan, H. (1982b). The impact of hearing impairment and the need to facilitate adjustment. In R. H. Hull (Ed.), *Rehabilitative audiology* (pp. 69-80). New York: Grune and Stratton.

Kasden, S. (1970). Speech discrimination in two age groups matched for hearing loss. *Journal of Auditory Research, 10,* 210-212.

Kirikae, I. (1969). Auditory function in advanced age with reference to histological changes in the central auditory system. *International Audiology, 8,* 221-230.

Lovering, L. J., and Hardick, E. J. (1969). Lipreading performance as a function of visual acuity. Paper presented at the Annual Meeting of the American Speech and Hearing Association, Chicago.

Maurer, J. F., and Rupp, R. R. (1979). *Hearing and aging* (pp. 33-66, 96-178). New York: Grune and Stratton.

McCarthy, P. A., and Alpiner, J. G. (1978). The remediation process. In J. G. Alpiner (Ed.), *Handbook of adult rehabilitative audiology* (pp. 88-120). Baltimore: Williams and Wilkins.

Nitchie, E. G. (1930). *Lipreading: Principles and practice.* (p. 341). New York: Lippincott.

Noble, W. G. (1978). *Assessment of impaired hearing: A critique and a new method* (pp. 264-269). New York: Academic Press.

Noble, W. G., and Atherly, G. (1970). The hearing measurement scale: A questionnaire for the assessment of auditory disability. *Journal of Auditory Research, 10,* 229-250.

O'Neill, J. J., and Oyer, H. J. (1981). *Visual communication for the hard of hearing.* Englewood Cliffs, NJ: Prentice-Hall.

Orchik, D. J., and Burgess, J. (1977). Synthetic sentence identification as a function of the age of the listener. *Journal of the American Auditory Society, 3,* 42-46.

Pelson, R. O., and Prather, W. F. (1974). Effects of visual message-related cues: Age and hearing impairment on speech-reading performance. *Journal of Speech and Hearing Research, 17,* 518-525.

Pestalozza, G., and Shore, I. (1955). Clinical evaluation of presbycusis on the basis of different tests of auditory function. *Laryngoscope, 65,* 1136-1163.

Popelka, G. R., and Berger, K. W. (1971). Gestures and speech reception. *American Annals of the Deaf, 116,* 434-436.

Riegel, K. (1956). A study of verbal achievement of older persons. *Journal of Gerontology, 14,* 453-456.

Rupp, R. R., and Heavenrich, A. Z. (1982). Positive communication game rules. Parts 1, 2, and 3. *Hearing Instruments, 33,* 34 and 64, 16-19, 20-22.

Rupp, R., Higgins, J., and Maurer, J. (1977). A feasibility scale for predicting hearing aid use (FSPHAU) with older individuals. *Journal of the Academy of Rehabilitative Audiology, 10,* 81-104.

Schow, R. L., Christensen, J. M., Hutchinson, J. M., and Nerbonne, M. A. (1978). *Communication disorders of the aged.* Baltimore: University Park Press.

Schuknecht, H. (1955). Presbycusis. *Laryngoscope, 65,* 402-419.

Schuknecht, H. (1964). Further observations on the pathology of presbycusis. *Archives of Otolaryngology, 80,* 369-382.

Shoop, C., and Binnie, C. A. (1978). The effect of age on the visual perception of speech. *Scandinavian Audiology, 7,* 3-8.

Simmons, A. A. (1959). Factors related to lipreading. *Journal of Speech and Hearing Research, 2,* 340-353.

Smith, R., and Prather, W. (1971). Phoneme discrimination in older persons under varying signal-to-noise conditions. *Journal of Speech and Hearing Research, 14,* 630-638.

Stone, L. (1957). Facial cues of context in lip reading. In E. I. Lowell (Ed.), *John Tracy Clinic research papers* (Vol. 5). Los Angeles: John Tracy Clinic.

Vaughn, G. R., Lightfoot, R. K., and Gibbs, S. D. (1983). Assistive listening devices: Space. *ASHA, 25*(3), 33-46.

Ventry, I., and Weinstein, B. (1982). Hearing handicap inventory for the elderly. (HHIE). *Ear and Hearing, 3*(3), 128-134.

Wallace, J. (1956). Some studies of perception in relation to age. *British Journal of Psychology, 47,* 283-297.

Wax, T. (1982). The hearing impaired aged: Double jeopardy. *Gallaudet Today, 12,* 3-7.

Chapter 7
The Psychology of Hearing Loss

Hilde S. Schlesinger

Simone de Beauvoir knows that in old age, the well-to-do fare better than the needy. It is clear that the age at which decline begins has always depended on the class one belongs to. Today a miner is finished at 50, whereas among the privileged, many carry their years with ease . . . .

It is the fault of society that the decline of age begins prematurely and is precipitous, physically painful and morally terrifying—because people come to it with empty hands. (Parenti, 1978, p. 68)

Fling the emptiness out of your arms (Rainer Maria Rilke)

REACTIONS TO AGING

Different life experiences can lead to a similar "psychology." Such disparate groups as the elderly, the poor, women, members of minority groups and the disabled, for example, often share a sense of powerlessness and all its critical consequences. A causal circle has been hypothesized and will be illustrated with emphasis on aging and hearing loss.

"Aging" has different meanings to different persons. It is seen as both a positive and a negative process: a growth and a decline (Birren, Imus, and Windle, 1959; Gottlieb, 1983). Some see only the negative, the loss of self-esteem, the weakness, scarce supplies and increasing threats to security (Busse, 1965, p. 81). Lindbergh (1955, p. 87) suggests, "This period of expanding is often tragically misunderstood . . . . The signs that presage growth, so similar . . . to those in early adolescence: discontent, restlessness, doubt, despair, longing, are interpreted falsely as signs of decay."

The author wishes to thank Catherine Borchert for her creative library research, Iris Daigre for her untiring effort and support, and Katherine Chamberlin for her kind editing assistance.

The word "aging" may be appropriate for the biological system, but "changing" is more accurate for interpersonal, cultural, economic, and systems. other Those who "fight the system" may outlive those who "age gracefully" (Haak, 1976, pp. 23-24). Indeed, grace may be the result of passivity and not of Erikson's genuine serenity.

As Posner (1982, p. 50) indicates, higher neurological functions are to a great degree preserved in normal older people. Verbal intelligence seems to increase year by year so that healthy 80 year olds do better than college seniors at verbal intelligence tests. "Learned abilities increased over time for adults of all ages, while biologically based abilities declined for all adults over 40. There is no decrement in learned abilities, and the decline in overall ability is due to a general functional decline within the central nervous system" (Nesselroade, Schaie, and Baltes, 1972, p. 224).

In general, both creativity and abstract problem solving is influenced by many cultural, educational, and social factors (Atchley, 1983, p. 62). For example, "the self esteem scores of older people living *independently* in the community are nearly double those of high school students" (Atchley, 1983, p. 79). On the other hand, a group being considered for admission to a retirement home had "more latent pathology than did elderly subjects remaining in the community" (Busse, 1965, p. 85).

The elderly are vulnerable to the loss of friends, jobs, transportation, and entertainment. Each needs to cope with the terrible "prey of boredom even if he preserves his health and mental faculties. Deprived of his grip on the world, he is unable to regain it because apart from work his leisure was alienated" (de Beauvoir, cited in Parenti, 1978, p. 68). The numbers who have succumbed to losses may be exaggerated; according to one report, in 1977 "84 per cent of people 55 and over had no major activity limitation and 90 per cent had adequate transportation" (Atchley, 1983, p. 109).

However, there are more somber notes. Often, "preservatives are offered or self-utilized . . . rather than any inner transformation that would permit self renewal" (Riesman, quoted in Zetzel, 1965, p. 119). The elderly in America do not enjoy the deference offered in more traditional societies, but are treated with "impatience, patronization and finally incarceration in a nursing home. As the elderly are given more years to live, they are given less reason to live" (Parenti, 1978, p. 68).

The Chinese psychiatrist Wu Chen-I believes that depression in the elderly is more prevalent in the West. "Much has been said of our Western tendency to extrude older citizens from the bosom of society. They lose their place in the family, in industry, and in the community, and as their *sphere of influence is eroded*, their morale collapses, leaving them vulnerable to disability and disease" (Greenblatt and Chien, 1983, p. 206).

Others attribute more causal force to early environmental vicissitudes. A gamut of symptoms associated with increasing demands on the environment, but not necessarily with depression, is a common clinical picture. "It is a neurosis common in later years of life, and determined by early failures which may remain latent while immature, excessive needs are met by gratifying life situations" (Zetzel, 1965, p. 117). The World Health Organization (1959, pp. 24-29) gives credence to the "continuity" of pathology and indicates that one half of persons with affective illnesses have morbidity and pathology prior to age 60. Similarly, paraphrenics ("Mais où sont les neiges d'antan?") are said to have been ill for 10 or 20 years. Some 30 or 40 per cent of them also show severe visual and auditory impairment.

Elderly people are often called "crocks" (Zarit, 1980, p. 87). They are often ill, poor, without resources, and surrounded by people who avoid them. Physiological, parental, and societal factors all play a part. Elderly people have been judged to be conservative, cautious, rigid, and uncertain. Research, however, has found both rigidity and cautiousness to be multifactorial and not present in the elderly to a particularly high degree. Cautiousness is reported for both answering and *hearing* (Zarit, 1980, p. 61). One explanation for the "conservatism" of today's elderly may be that when young they were already more conservative than the youth of today. Gelfand (1982, p. 31) finds the cautiousness of this "first generation of Americans who had struggled to attain a sense of security in their old age" perfectly understandable. Elderly members of ethnic minority groups have lived through events well-designed to provoke caution. "Second and third generation elderly people with less troubled history may be more assertive . . . ."

One study compared discourse samples of ten young adults (mean age, 23) and ten elderly adults (mean age, 80) for frequency of "uncertainty" behaviors (revisions, hesitant interjections and fillers, unfinished utterances not revised, and number of prompts by the examiner), frequency and location of pauses, and various utterance length characteristics. The older subjects differed from the younger only in their more hesitant interjections and fillers (Gordon and colleagues, quoted in Schow, Christensen, Hutchinson, and Nerbonne, 1980, p. 98). The elderly may be hesitant if their own communications are frequently disregarded and dismissed.

However, the prevalence of mental illness is highest during the last decades of life: "18 to 25 percent of old people experienced diminution of their mental health. It appears that depression is the lot of one in four persons aged over 60" (Hovaguimian, 1982, pp. 30-31).

GROWING OLD AND BECOMING DEAF

Glass (1983, pp. 3-5) observes that elderly persons process auditory cues more slowly and in a different sequence. As sleep apnea increases with age, "micro-units of undetectable cochlear damage might occur during the sleep apnea of elderly people." She notes the paucity of information about the interaction of multiple drugs on hearing loss.

Posner (1982, p. 49) points out that decreased renal function affects the action of antibiotics in older patients. Furthermore, the ototoxicity of certain antibiotics is increased when diuretics are prescribed to older patients. The elderly and the victims of "orphan" illnesses may develop a feeling of powerlessness when their problems are not considered important enough to warrant attention and research.

What, if any, additional problems are caused by the combination of aging and deafness? Old age is vastly different for those who were deaf as children than for those who became deaf in later life. As Schein (1984) has maintained movingly and as Becker (1980) observed, the former have a support system, the deaf community, that stands them in good stead throughout their life. As with other groups, those who have suffered from prejudice, whose language, ethnicity, or disability has been derogated early, find themselves later in less contact with the majority culture, and establish or gain a new sense of community, *power*, and competence.

Schow and Nerbonne (1982, p. 142) constructed a questionnaire for hard-of-hearing adults, incorporating both audiometric and non-audiometric assessment. Ventry and Weinstein (1982, pp. 128-134) also used a questionnaire for the self-assessment of emotional and social adjustment by hearing impaired, elderly individuals. Both studies found a great range in the degree of adjustment to hearing impairment.

McCroskey and Kasten (1982, pp. 124-125) describe increased auditory fusion (the inability to detect short, silent intervals between acoustic events). Altered speech rates (particularly slowing) improve the speech perception of elderly individuals. A combination of body and soul may be at work here, since a slower speaker usually looks more attentive and interested. Eisdorfer (1960) stated that elderly persons with impaired hearing or vision were more likely than those with normal senses to exhibit an overcontrolled, withdrawn, or rigid personality. Powers and Powers (1978), in a study involving 226 subjects, found little difference in social involvement between those with and without hearing loss, except for an increased contact with children by the former. Norris and Cunningham (1981) found that increased hearing loss decreased social activities planned by others but increased other social activities.

Cooper (1979, p. 422) has reversed himself and now states that, "thus far, studies of personality traits in the hard-of-hearing have failed to reveal consistent patterns of abnormality . . . that would predispose to psychotic, particularly schizophrenic, breakdown." Singerman, Riedner, and Folstein (1980, p. 62) demonstrated that a substantial proportion of audiological outpatients were at risk for psychiatric morbidity. The psychiatric casualties occurred when the patients had no associated hearing loss but solely otologic problems.

Alpiner (1978, pp. 171-174) suggests that many factors—health, housing, transportation, nutrition, hearing, age—are important to the adjustment of the elderly, but the most "important consideration is the need to create a psychological attitude that negates the hopelessness [powerlessness] of feeling old . . . . Persons living in confined environments appeared to exhibit considerably greater difficulty in overcoming their handicaps."

In an investigation of paranoid reactions in normal college students experiencing a temporary hearing loss induced by hypnosis, support was found for "a hypothesized cognitive-social mechanism for the clinically observable relationship between paranoia and deafness in the elderly" (Zimbardo, Andersen, and Kabat, 1981, p. 1531). Zarit (1980) speculates that paranoid symptoms often have obvious functions such as alleviating isolation by calling helping agencies to one's aid, accounting for the weakness and attributing it to others' malevolence, and supplying stimuli lost with the sensory loss. Attention for appropriate behavior may diminish the need for "attention getting maneuvers" (p. 219).

Von der Lieth (1972) reports three main findings during his self-induced deafness: the withdrawal of others, inability to engage in group communication, and the necessity of interrupting the experiment during a family crisis—something a deaf person cannot do. M. Nguyen (personal communication, 1984) has been investigating the relationship between compliance with medical and audiological referral and the process of denial in a population suffering from hearing loss.

Many have commented on the isolation, loneliness, and withdrawal accompanying deafness and aging. Pieces of the puzzle relating the variable of power or powerlessness to the impact of aging and hearing loss are beginning to fit together.

DEFINITIONS OF POWER

There are innumerable definitions of power; interestingly, most do not imply an intent to constrain other people, but a sensed ability to influence and control the environment.

"The concept of power has an elusive, almost intangible quality" [Kaufman and Jones, 1954, p. 205]. Yet for all its elusiveness the concept . . . remains irresistible. Just as soon as some social scientists decide to discard it, out of suspicion that it raises too many semantic problems, "power" creeps back into their pages wearing such disguises as "influence," "control," "dominance" and so forth. When a concept continues to prove so troublesome, yet so compelling, it is usually because it refers to phenomena that crave explanation. And whereas we may dismiss the term as bothersome, this does not satisfy the craving. (Parenti, 1978, p. 3)

To McClelland (1975), power is the need to have impact, establishing, maintaining, or restoring prestige or reputation. Power can be achieved by strong action, assaults, and aggression; by help, assistance, or advice; by actions that produce emotions in others; and by a concern for reputation.

May (1979, pp. 142-143) remarks that " . . . the original meaning of the word power (its original stem in Latin) is 'posse' which means 'I can and I will.' This is significant because the acquisition of power, the power within one's self and the awareness that one can influence other people, is essential to . . . confidence and mental health . . . ."

Parenti (1978, pp. 63-68) notes that power and powerlessness are relative and contextual. He considers certain groups with little power: those at the bottom of the economic ladder, with little control over the conditions of their lives. "The disadvantages suffered by other categories of people, such as the very young, the very old, women, ethnic minorities, and those who are 'institutionalized' for physical and presumably mental disabilities are greatly compounded by class position and are . . . partly a function of class." The experience of powerlessness, Goldenberg (1978, p. 42) states, is perhaps the single most important common feature of oppressed people. Janeway (1980, p. 49) observes that "the way that children learn to understand and exercise ordered uses of power within relationships is a central part of normal growth, the primary and the earliest fashion in which the individual becomes involved in society." She discusses the profound disorders of power that "affect the very root of personality: the capacity to assert one's will by choosing between 'yes' and 'no'; the daring that can commit emotion purposefully to a future goal, the sheer physical control of nerve and muscle and the steady mental effort which teaches the competence that Erikson sees as the goal of the next step in growth and trust."

Several authors have investigated the role of "perceived" control in human functioning. Research has shown that actual control is not as important as the belief, true or not, that, if one wanted to, one could exercise control in a given situation. If this is the case, it would be crucial to investigate groups, such as the elderly, who characteristically have been denied the opportunity to exercise control. In an experiment reported by Langer (1981, p. 256), one group of nursing home residents was told that "they were fully capable of making decisions and . . . *should* continue to make all the decisions previously made independently . . . .They were also given a plant to take care of." A second group was told that the staff were eager to help them (with the implication that they had decreased competence) and would look after the plants they were given. At the outset, both groups were comparable in socioeconomic status and in physical and mental health. After 18 months, the first group was significantly more alert, happily active, and well, and fewer had died (Langer and Rodin, 1976; Rodin and Langer, 1977).

The perception of a loss of control may disrupt normal functioning; when control is reinstated, normal functioning may be restored. The helplessness literature started by Seligman (1975; Garber and Seligman, 1980) indicates that, with a lasting inability to avoid negative outcomes, individuals give up and become passive. Generalizing from these uncontrollable situations to others that are, in fact, controllable, they develop an *illusion of incompetence*. Occasionally, an *illusion of control* arises when individuals engaging in chance behaviors, such as gambling, act as if they had control and were practicing a skill. Many behaviors occur *mindlessly* and sometimes, in normal environments, such mindlessness can be adaptive. However, in nursing homes the environment is so unvarying that there is little need for active, conscious, cognitive work. Reduced information processing is noxious to the elderly individual (Langer, 1981, p. 270).

Most of us exercise some kind of power in one situation or another, but no one is all-powerful in all things. Even children, the frail elderly, and the severely disabled can achieve a sense of power in a supportive social network. However, changes in dialogue between mothers and their children or helpers and "helpees" can lead to lowered autonomy and performance in the children and the aged.

THE THEORY OF POWERLESSNESS, DIALOGUE, AND EARLY DEVELOPMENT

Too many deaf children and adults and too many disabled and disadvantaged individuals share certain characteristics such as immaturity, impulsivity, spatial versus temporal orientation, and attention to the "here and now" and not to the future. These groups also lag behind academic and vocational norms despite normal intellectual potential (Altshuler, 1964; Altshuler, Deming, Vollenweider, Rainer, and Tendler, 1976; Auletta, 1981; Greenspan, 1981; Levine, 1956; Sadock, Kaplan, Freedman, and Sussman, 1975; Sherman and Robinson, 1982).

It is postulated that these similarities are engendered by specific parental experiences leading to psychological stances of powerlessness. It has been said that when social scientists describe a large group of disadvantaged individuals, they describe the psychological consequences of powerlessness (Haggstrom, 1964).

"Powerlessness," as used in this chapter, signifies an individual's self-perception as not having the cognitive competence, psychological skills, instrumental resources, and support systems needed to influence his or her environment successfully. "Surplus powerlessness . . . cripples people and makes them believe that they cannot change; it allows people to interpret their victories merely as defeats, to be pessimistic about what they can accomplish, cynical about whom they can trust and hence reluctant to define tasks and goals for themselves.... The sources of this powerlessness reside in childhood socialization and are reinforced by the powerlessness experienced in adult life" (Lerner, 1979, p. 19).

Although the sources of powerlessness differ, the effect on mother-child interaction is similar. Parents who feel powerful are more likely to grant and demand autonomy and to behave in relatively egalitarian terms. They describe desirable qualities of the child as happiness, considerateness, curiosity, and self-control. Less powerful parents tend to have excessive contact, to be controlling, intrusive, punitive, and irritable, and to consider neatness, cleanliness, and obedience desirable (Bronfenbrenner, 1958). One measurable outcome of powerlessness in parents is a tendency to "control." Barsch (1968) demonstrated that mothers of children identified as deficient or "different" adopt authoritarian attitudes; they become directive and critical, and tend to interfere with and structure change for their children. Research evidence indicates that parents of deaf children are more controlling and intrusive than parents of hearing children (Schlesinger and Meadow, 1972; Collins, 1969; Greenberg, 1980; Brinich, 1980; Schlesinger and Acree, 1984).

Children who are "different" have parents who are more controlling; are other sets of parents also more controlling? Does more "controlling" relate to parental powerlessness? Disadvantaged parents are more controlling and are seen as powerless by others and themselves. We postulate that parents who feel powerless are more likely to seek to "control" rather than to "elicit communication with" their child as described for mothers in general (Newport, Gleitman, and Gleitman, 1977; Snow, 1977; McDonald and Pien, 1982). One approach leads the child into dialogue, the other into avoidance of communication with parents and, later, with all adults, especially those in authority.

Schachter (1979) found that advantaged mothers more frequently engaged in dialogue *with* their child, whereas disadvantaged mothers more frequently talked *at* their child. The advantaged mothers used "control talk" half as often and gave justifications for their "do's, don'ts, and refusals" twice as often as the disadvantaged mothers. Overall, advantaged parents "appear to support and facilitate the actions of their toddlers." Evidently parents who feel in adequate control of their lives are freer to support the autonomous action of their toddlers. Parental support, in turn, can enhance the child's self confidence, sense of mastery, and power, which affect his motivation and performance in linguistic and cognitive tasks. The powerless, disadvantaged parents, on the other hand, have difficulty supporting their toddlers when they begin to assert their power.

Evidence is accumulating (Borchert and Daigre, 1984; Schlesinger and Acree, 1984) that the dialogue stances of parents of "communicatively successful and unsuccessful" deaf children resemble those of advantaged and disadvantaged parents. For example, the mothers of the communicatively successful youngsters in the study by Schlesinger and Acree (1984) engaged in more responsive and less command talk, and repeated the child's speech more often than did the mothers of the less successful youngsters, who talked *at* their children, gave more commands, and repeated themselves more often. The frustration stemming from unproductive interactions is widely known.

The language differences between disadvantaged and advantaged youngsters and the different communicative styles of their mothers resemble the differences between elderly nursing home residents and old people functioning within a community. One group receives a stream of advice, help, and orders; the other is engaged in egalitarian dialogue.

Such early language interactions, the feelings associated with them, and their affective and motivational consequences may be key factors in disadvantaged children's poor performance on school tasks and tests. These factors have been identified as low self-esteem, low effectance motivation, and wariness of adults (Zigler and Butterfield, 1968; Zigler and Trickett, 1978).

It is plausible and adaptive for children who were talked at rather than with and who heard many imperatives and prohibitions from their powerless parents to shun dialogue with adults. Indeed, disadvantaged, deaf children with hearing parents are said to learn language primarily from their peers.

Some language functions that differentiate advantaged from disadvantaged toddlers can also be explained by the powerlessness theory. The diminished use of the future tense may be associated with a diminished sense of future hope. The future is unimportant to those who feel powerless, for if they cannot influence or control it, they grow fatalistic, as the disadvantaged so often do. And if they cannot influence others, they do not learn, and they grow weary of adopting the perspective of others. Powerlessness can lead to non-ego-syntonic power strategies such as dawdling, eye avoidance, obsessive manipulation of the physical environment, dialogue reticence, or exaggerated talkativeness. General opposition to society may develop, especially in authority relationships.

The theory of the consequences of powerlessness is applicable to other disabilities. Similar trends are exhibited by the mothers of blind, hyperactive, and orthopedically handicapped children, as similar behaviors and achievements are attained by the children (Carpignano, 1984; Kekelis, 1981; Lambert, Sandoval, and Sassone, 1978). The theory is applicable to anyone, at any age, who develops a temporary or permanent feeling of helplessness (Seligman, 1975). Powerless, helpless individuals may withdraw from human contact or develop such imperative, demanding, and controlling stances that others withdraw from them, thus aggravating their original sense of helplessness. The parallels with aged, deafened individuals are apparent.

This unfortunate but reversible cycle of maternal monologue, child communicative reticence, low motivational stances in school, and low school performance started with parental powerlessness in many disparate groups. How can the sources and results of powerlessness be so similar in such different groups?

Disadvantaged parents feel powerless because of their low status in society and their dependence on others for basic life support (Slaughter, 1970). Disadvantaged mothers see themselves as powerless, helpless, and unable to influence the development of their children (Minuchin, Montalva, Guerney, Fosman, and Schumer, 1967). The parents of disabled children, on the other hand, feel powerless because their usual practices do not result in the behavior they expect from the child. When deep memories of what children do (turn to, smile at, and *understand* their voice) are not confirmed, the parents are perplexed, and their perplexity is in some way conveyed to the child.

Since, despite the dire examples mentioned above, some splendid human beings emerge from powerless and vulnerable groups, some munificence, some benevolence, some grace protects them. In part, that grace appears magical; in part, it rests on the support, warmth, and respect of others.

OTHER DIALOGUE STANCES RELATED TO POWERLESSNESS

Having noted that powerlessness evokes certain communicative styles between mothers and children, let us consider dialogue relations between any two people under certain circumstances. Fowler and Kress (1979, p. 185) note that there are "strong and pervasive connections between linguistic structure and social structure." The researchers Halliday (1975) and Harris (1983) suggest that language ability and communicative competence are a product of social structure. One factor that recurs in many studies of sociolinguistic variation is status or power, and differences in power. This is explicit in Brown and Gilman's (1972) famous paper "The Pronouns of Power and Solidarity," in which they contend that "Prominent among the social structures which influence linguistic structures is inequality of power.... Language not only encodes power differences but is instrumental in enforcing them."

Oyer (1976, p. 50) gives interesting examples of variables influencing communication. Semantic aspects of language that change over generations influence communication between parents and children. Fatigue can interfere with communication and produce the picture of disinterest, passivity, or even senility. On the other hand, speaking with persons who have sustained a hearing loss requires extra expenditures of energy. After interviewing women who had sustained a hearing loss, Oyer was noticeably fatigued. Such fatigue imposes stress on friends and family members and can contribute to the isolation of hard-of-hearing persons. Oyer and Paolucci (1970) found, for example, that the husbands of homemakers with severe hearing losses scored high on a test of marital tension.

Another study indicates that the older family member with a hearing and speech deficit that makes communication difficult is more likely to be placed in a nursing home by his family than is the incontinent or bedridden elderly person (Elconin et al., cited in Schow et al., 1980, p. 306).

The aged, the disabled, and the aged deaf are often seen as individuals to be avoided (Dunkel-Schetter and Wortman, 1981, pp. 366-368). Resident patients interviewed in a long-term care facility said "that at least an average amount of communication was occurring around them, but that they themselves spoke very little." The content and functions of the patients' communications were extremely basic, with relatively few socially directed statements (Lubinski, Morrison, and Rigrodsky, 1981).

How do dialogue stances between parents and young children resemble other dialogue situations? In my early experience, much patience and creativity was necessary to establish a meaningful dialogue with deafened patients. Initially, I spoke more and not responsively. Out of powerlessness and inability to engage the patients in a genuine exchange, I made more suggestions and used more attention-getting devices. Upon first entering my office, one patient exclaimed, "I was never a happy hearing woman; your task is to make me a happy deaf woman." She then sat down and engaged in visual avoidance and other control maneuvers. Attention-getting devices on my part provoked communicational reticence or barrage, not a genuine dialogue. It took a few weeks to recover my equilibrium and a few months before the patient settled down to mourn her loss, plan for, and discuss her future.

Another patient, a troubled youth before the onset of deafness, refused to look, to accept written communication, or to learn sign language. He reminded me of the classic psychoanalytic case of a young black boy of yesteryear who sat in the playroom for months with his feet on the desk. Eventually, he smiled and asked the therapist, "Do you know that I am playing white man?" My patient felt powerless in all areas: health, the ability to drive, and a total absence of plans for the future, for work, school, or play. He desperately needed a renewed sense of power.

A third patient refused paper communication, although his lipreading skills were not adequate for dialogue, and said that others avoided him.

"They cannot cope with my deafness and refuse to deal with me at all, figuring that I am window dressing for hiring the handicapped . . . . My word is seldom acceptable." His comments were depressed and hopeless.

However, a deafened man 60 years of age was constructive and serene. He sketched his physicians and medical procedures, constructed beautiful objets d'art, and found countless ways to communicate with friends or anyone who crossed his path. In no way did that Puckish character succumb to powerlessness.

After the initial mourning crisis, psychological reactions to hearing loss are primarily contextual. The deafened persons I have described, and others I have known as friends and colleagues, had vastly different personalities. As Meadow indicated (1980), there is nothing inherent in early onset deafness that should produce the psychological problems we observe. Nor need late onset deafness damage human relationships and dialogue, and frequently it does not. Some adults withdraw; some, deaf or hearing, behave like children with their families and caretakers. They may behave like the youngster described by Janeway (1980, pp. 55-56). "George had great power over his family. They allowed him to exercise his random gusts of willingness, they bought him out of scrapes . . . . But all this did George no good. License was granted to him, but not as a part of a continuing process of interaction between equals, interaction that held him responsible for what he did. And therefore he was not given validation for his actions, he was still a nothing. He could do anything—but the price was that what he did had no meaning." Some adults, young and old, hearing and deaf alike, make incessant shrill demands; nothing really satisfies them. Such behavior reflects a deep sense of narcissistic incompetence and powerlessness.

THE HELPING PROCESS

> Good can't be done to people unless they are allowed to have a stake in choosing the good and effectuating the doing. (Janeway, 1980, p. 57)

"Help is usually given in the hope that it will do some good . . . . It would then follow that potential donors of help would be . . . disturbed by the prospect that their help will not only fail, but actually leave the recipient worse off. Yet there is strong evidence that well meaning helpers may often do more harm than good" (Coates, Renzaglia, and Embree [1983], quoted in Staff, Institute for Information Studies, 1983). "A large portion of what comprises social support consists of rendering help or assistance to the ill [aged, or disabled] person. It is commonly assumed that the recipients of this assistance will be appreciative of the donor" (Suls, 1982, p. 271). The helpee, however, often exhibits "feelings of tension and obligation, decrements in self-esteem and social status, and derogation of the helper, and the help" (Fisher, De Paulo, and Nadler, 1981, p. 368). The "thank you's" forced from a poor child's mouth to a rich lady bountiful can produce long-standing fury. After World War II, European recipients of Marshall Plan aid frequently denigrated the help and the helpers.

Service providers tend to attribute two types of responsibility to the individuals whom they help. Causal responsibility is attributed when the helpers believe that people *could* produce certain outcomes, whereas moral responsibility is attributed to helpees who *should* produce given outcomes. Apparently the latter is more important to helpers. At least four models of helping can be identified as related to moral responsibility, each associated with a different orientation to the world, each internally coherent, and each in some measure incompatible with the other three (Brickman et al., 1982, p. 369).

In the Moral Model, individuals are responsible for both their problems and their solutions. "You are the master of your fate, you are the captain of your soul" (Henley, 1894). The author, said to be disabled, probably had extensive contact with helping professionals. In this model, no one needs to help since each individual manufactures his or her troubles, and no one can help since all must find their own solution. The model impels people to change or to stop complaining. Those who cannot or will not do either, may become pathologically lonely.

In the Compensatory Model, people are not blamed for their problems but are held responsible for solving them. This model impels action, often collaborative, and gives credit and respect to those who overcome their problems. It can, however, produce excessive striving for achievement, competition, and control. Hostility is provoked when strivings are thwarted, and there may be a greater vulnerability to heart attacks.

The Enlightenment Model holds people responsible for problems, but not solutions, and leads them to accept "a strikingly negative image of themselves and . . . a strong degree of submission to agents of social control . . . ." This model can lead to a fanatic or obsessive concern with certain problems and place unwarranted power in agents of social change or control.

The Medical Model holds people responsible for neither problems nor solutions. They are to see themselves, and are seen by others, as ill or incapacitated. This model fosters dependency and incompetence. Indeed, Wack and Rodin argue that much of the helplessness of nursing home residents can be traced directly to medical procedures (Brickman et al., 1982, p. 373).

Coates and colleagues (1983) note the "unfortunate irony" that giving help "can reduce both the actual and perceived capabilities of recipients, and thereby render them helpless." Help may be so overwhelming as to reduce the sense of control, hinder the maintenance and acquisition of new skills, and undermine self-esteem and competence. The sense of control may also be undermined by creating confusion about the attribution of credit or blame for the outcome of any action. Depressed people tend to give credit to others, which does not bolster mental health.

THE HELPING PROCESS AND ELDERLY, DEAFENED INDIVIDUALS

Deafened, elderly individuals are often disinterested in the help and advice of audiologists. This disinterest is so intense and universal that clinics try everything but "dancing girls" to overcome it (Alpiner, quoted in Schow et al., 1980, p. 305). Such a disinterest in, or rebellion against, help may promote a fictitious sense of power.

Audiologists often complain that their advice is disregarded. Many hearing problems persist among elderly nursing home residents (Schow et al., 1980) who are reluctant to seek care, use aids, or admit their loss. In one case, 5 of 8 nursing home residents refused free hearing aids (Gaitz and Warshaw, 1964). In another, only 6 of 48 residents referred for evaluation followed advice (Alpiner, cited in Schow et al., p. 312). Resisting or refusing to wear a hearing aid in nursing homes may represent an unwillingness to adjust to a new, strange environment. At the same time, patients may use their hearing loss as an excuse for decreased participation in social activities. The move into a nursing home signifies a loss of freedom and independence as well as impending death (Rosenwasser, 1964).

What might provoke compliance or refusal? Johnson (1982, p. 94) emphasizes the "importance of assessing the patient's motivation to use hearing aids . . . . Some elderly individuals . . . are said to prefer the relative quiet of their world to the sounds heard through a hearing aid." Hardick (1977, pp. 323-324) writes that the hearing-impaired elderly have to be sold on the benefits of hearing again. Both authors suggest that the elderly prefer "peace and quiet," but this preference may stem from a wish to shut off painful dialogues and monologues perceived as unresponsive to their needs.

Aural rehabilitation programs recommend a hearing aid evaluation and orientation; counseling of client and family; communication rehabilitation, including auditory training and speechreading; and comprehensive planning for emotional, social, and vocational adjustment (Schow et al., 1980, p. 307). Specific communication techniques are also recommended, such as good lighting, low reverberation, high signal-to-noise ratio, expertise in interacting with conversational partners, better listening skills, and skills to deal with the impatient hearing person. But why the frequent failures? These, we postulate, are related to the sense of powerlessness.

THE HELPERS AND THE SOCIAL NETWORK

Supportive environments can reverse the vicious circle of powerlessness and its effect on communicative stances. Effective individual or group support is not coercive or controlling and does not consist of didactic lessons and advice (Gottlieb, 1983). Children and parents who *dialogue* effectively and with delight feel more powerful. Their interchanges are marked by a greater sense of mastery and less need for control, and their parents are able to pursue linguistic and psychological strategies that foster the child's autonomy and motivation to learn.

Helpers of the powerless develop fatigue, exasperation, and avoidance techniques or overinvolvement and burnout (Maslach, 1982). Dunkel-Schetter and Wortman (1981) suggest that the elderly often fail to receive support because their suffering evokes feelings of vulnerability, helplessness, and incompetence in potential helpers. The parallels to elderly deafened individuals and their helpers are clear. Luey (1980, p. 254) describes the plight of the social worker helping the hearing impaired. When normal communicative behavior fails, dialogue can break down and the client may "demand repetition, may simply look pained and frustrated, or may nod politely and then reveal his lack of understanding with inappropriate responses. The social worker may not understand the reasons for these difficulties . . . . Mutual frustration is inevitable. A social worker in such a situation is likely to feel helpless."

SUMMARY

Psychological responses to hearing loss in adulthood are crucially influenced by prior psychological development, the sense of power during childhood and adulthood, the degree and rapidity of the loss of power at the time of hearing loss, and the investment in language and communication versus other ego functions. They are further influenced by the level of helplessness created in the family and helpers, the ability to provide *responsive communication*, and the support systems available to the newly deafened individual, his family, and helpers. These include a relative freedom from financial worries, good health and access to health professionals, physical mobility, and perceived encouragement for personal interests and activities. Support comes from ongoing, consistent contact and dialogue with, and interest and respect from, others.

CONCLUSIONS

The so-called "Psychology of deafness" is less related to the nature of the disability than to its meaning to the individual. The lost dream matters more than the extent of the sensory loss.

Frankel and Turner (1983) studied 420 Canadian adults whose hearing was impaired after the age of 15. All were tested for hearing impairment, communication handicap, psychological distress, and social support. The degree of psychological distress was more closely related to the level of the social support and the experience of the handicap than to the degree of impairment (p. 285). Similarly, Stahlecker (in press), studying neurologically impaired or developmentally disabled infants, found no relation between the *degree* of a child's impairment and the quality of the mother's attachment. However, the mother's experience of the handicap—the difference between her dream and her reality—was significant.

The psychology of hearing loss is contextual and multifactorial, and the differences between *the dream and the reality* are vital. Deafened, elderly persons are not psychologically homogeneous and the sources of their heterogeneity must be elucidated. Understanding these sources may help us to promote the "period of expanding... [and] growth" (Lindbergh, 1955, p. 87).

We can see powerful, moving, and serene "old" faces as beautiful and competent when they come from afar, from other cultures. We are beginning to regard the signing and the "voices" of the deaf as merely different, and *not* deficient. The elderly person's feelings of "emptiness" will be flung out when familiar old faces are seen as beautiful and competent and when the deafened person is regarded with patience and respect.

REFERENCES

Alpiner, J. G. (1978). Psychological and social aspects of aging as related to hearing rehabilitation of elderly clients. In M. A. Henoch (Ed.), *Aural rehabilitation for the elderly.* New York: Grune and Stratton.

Altshuler, K. Z. (1964). Personality traits and depressive symptoms in the deaf. In J. Wortis (Ed.), *Recent advances in biological psychiatry* (Vol. 6). New York: Plenum.

Altshuler, K. Z., Deming, W. E., Vollenweider, J., Rainer, J. D., and Tendler, R. (1976). Impulsivity and profound early deafness: A cross cultural inquiry. *American Annals of the Deaf, 131,* 331-345.

Atchley, R. C. (1983). *Aging: Continuity and change.* Belmont, CA: Wadsworth.

Auletta, K. (1968). *The underclass.* New York: Random House.

Barsch, R. H. (1968). *The parent of the handicapped child.* Springfield, IL: Charles C Thomas.

Becker, G. (1980). *Growing old in silence.* Berkeley: University of California.

Birren, J. E., Imus, H. A., and Windle, W. F. (1959). *The process of aging in the nervous system*. Springfield, IL: Charles C Thomas.

Borchert, C. M., and Daigre, I. (1983). *CAIRHI: Schachter scale modified for deaf toddlers*. Paper presented at Consortium on Human Dialogue, University of California, San Francisco.

Brickman, P., Rabinowitz, V. C., Karuza, J., Coates, D., Cohn, E., and Kidder, L. (1982). Models of helping and coping. *American Psychologist, 37*, 368-384.

Brinich, P. M. (1980). Childhood deafness and maternal control. *Journal of Communication Disorders, 13*, 75-81.

Bronfenbrenner, U. (1958). Socialization and social class through time and space. In E. E. Maccoby, T. M. Newcomb, and E. L. Hartley (Eds.), *Readings in social psychology*. New York: Holt, Rinehart and Winston.

Brown, R., and Gilman, A. (1972). The pronouns of power and solidarity. In P. P. Giglioli (Ed.), *Language and social context*. Harmondsworth: Penguin.

Busse, E. W. (1965). Research on aging: Some methods and findings. In M. A. Barezin and S. H. Cath (Eds.), *Geriatric Psychiatry*. New York: International Universities Press.

Carpignano, J. L. (1984). Effects of a role reversal model on the acquisition of labelling skills with orthopedically handicapped students. Unpublished manuscript.

Coates, D., Renzaglia, G., and Embree, M. (1983). When helping backfires: Help and helplessness. In J. D. Fisher and A. Nadler (Eds.), *New directions in helping. Vol. I. Recipient reactions to aid*. New York: Academic Press.

Collins, J. L. (1969). *Communication between deaf children of preschool age and their mothers*. (Doctoral dissertation, University of Pittsburgh). *Dissertation Abstracts International, 30*, 2245A.

Cooper, A. F. (1979). Deafness, psychiatric illness and the role of hearing loss in schizophrenia. In L. J. Bradford and W. G. Hardy (Eds.), Hearing and hearing impairment. New York: Grune and Stratton.

Dunkel-Schetter, C., and Wortman, C. B. (1981). Dilemmas of social support. In S. B. Kiesler, J. N. Morgan, and V. K. Oppenheimer (Eds.), *Aging: Social change*. New York: Academic Press.

Eisdorfer, C. (1960). Rorschach rigidity and sensory decrement in a senescent population. *Journal of Gerontology, 15*, 188-190.

Fisher, J. D., De Paulo, B. M., and Nadler, A. (1981). Extending altruism beyond the altruistic act. In J. P. Rushton and R. M. Sorrentino (Eds.), *Altruism and helping behavior*. Hillsdale, NJ: Lawrence Erlbaum Associates.

Fowler, R., and Kress, G. (1979). Critical linguistics. In R. Fowler, B. Hodge, G. Kress, and T. Trew (Eds.), *Language and control*. London: Routledge and Kegan Paul.

Frankel, B. G., and Turner, R. J. (1983). Psychological adjustment in chronic disability. *Canadian Journal of Sociology, 8*, 273-291.

Gaitz, C. M., and Warshaw, H. E. (1964). Obstacles encountered in correcting hearing loss in the elderly. *Geriatrics, 19*, 83-86.

Garber, J., and Seligman, M. E. P. (1980). *Human helplessness: Theory and applications*. New York: Academic Press.

Gelfand, D. E. (1982). *Aging: The ethnic factor*. Boston: Little, Brown.

Glass, L. (1983). *Hearing impairment and aging: Some research issues in the next decade*. Paper presented at the 9th World Congress of the World Federation of the Deaf, Palermo, Italy.

Goldenberg, I. I. (1978). *Oppression and social intervention*. Chicago: Nelson-Hall.

116   Schlesinger

Gottlieb, B. H. (1983). *Social support strategies*. Beverly Hills, CA: Sage Publications.

Greenberg, M. (1980). Social interaction between deaf preschoolers and their mothers. *Developmental Psychology, 16,* 465-474.

Greenblatt, M., and Chien, C. (1983). Depression in the elderly. In L. Breslau and M. Haug (Eds.), *Depression and aging: Causes, care, and consequences.* New York: Springer-Verlag.

Greenspan, S. I. (1981). *Psychopathology and adaptation in infancy and early childhood.* New York: International Universities Press.

Haak, L. A. (1976). A retiree's perspective on communication. In H. J. Oyer and E. J. Oyer (Eds.), *Aging and communication.* Baltimore: University Park Press.

Haggstrom, W. C. (1964). The power of the poor. In F. Riessman, J. Cohen, and A. Pearl (Eds.), *Mental health of the poor.* New York: Free Press.

Halliday, M. A. K. (1975). *Learning how to mean: Explanations in the development of language.* London: Arnold.

Hardick, E. J. (1977). Aural rehabilitation programs for the aged can be successful. *Journal of the Academy of Rehabilitative Audiology, 10,* 51-66.

Harris, A. (1983). Language and alienation. In B. Bain (Ed.), *Sociogenesis of language and human conduct.* New York: Plenum.

Henley, E. W. (1894). Invictus.

Hovaguimian, T. (1982). Mental health in old age. *World Health,* pp. 30-31.

Janeway, E. (1980). *Powers of the weak.* New York: Knopf.

Johnson, E. W. (1982). Hearing prostheses and communication aids for the elderly. *Medical Instrumentation, 16,* 93-94.

Kaufman, H., and Jones, V. (1954). The mystery of power. *Public Administration Review, 14,* 205.

Kekelis, L. S. (1981). *Mothers' input to blind children.* Unpublished master's thesis, University of Southern California, Los Angeles.

Lambert, N. M., Sandoval, J., and Sassone, D. (1978). Prevalence of hyperactivity in elementary school children as a function of social system definers. *American Journal of Orthopsychiatry, 48*(3), 446-463.

Langer, E. J. (1981). Old age: An artifact? In J. L. McGaugh and S. B. Kielser (Eds.), *Aging: Biology and behavior.* New York: Academic Press.

Langer, E. J., and Rodin, J. (1976). The effects of choice and enhanced personal responsibility for the aged. *Journal of Personality and Social Psychology, 37,* 2003-2013.

Lerner, M. (1979). Surplus powerlessness. *Social Policy, 9*(4), 11-27

Levine, E. S. (1956). *Youth in a soundless world.* New York: New York University.

Lindbergh, A. M. (1955). *Gift from the sea.* New York: Pantheon Books.

Lubinski, R., Morrison, E. B., and Rigrodsky, S. (1981). Perception of spoken communication by elderly chronically ill patients in an institutional setting. *Journal of Speech and Hearing Disorders, 46,* 405-412.

Luey, H. S. (1980). Between worlds: The problems of deafened adults. *Social Work in Health Care, 5,* 253-265.

Maslach, C. (1982). *Burnout: The cost of caring.* Englewood Cliffs, NJ: Prentice-Hall.

May, R. (1979). Psychoanalysis and power. In D. W. Harward (Ed.), *Power: Its nature, its use, its limits.* Boston: Schenkman.

McClelland, D. C. (1975). *Power: The inner experience.* New York: Irvington.

McCroskey, R. L., and Kasten, R. (1982). Temporal factors and the aging auditory system. *Ear and Hearing, 3,* 124-127.

McDonald, L., and Pien, D. (1982). Mother conversational behavior as a function of interactional intent. *Journal of Child Language, 9*, 337-358.

Meadow, K. P. (1980). *Deafness and child development.* Berkeley: University of California Press.

Minuchin, S., Montalva, B., Guerney, B. J., Fosman, B. L., and Schumer, F. L. (1967). *Families of the slums.* New York: Basic Books.

Nesselroade, J. R., Schaie, K. W., and Baltes, P. B. (1972). Ontogenetic and generational components of structural and quantitative change in adult behavior. *Journal of Gerontology, 27*(2), 222-228.

Newport, E., Gleitman, L., and Gleitman, H. (1977). Mother, I'd rather do it myself. In C. Ferguson and C. Snow (Eds.), *Talking to children.* London: Cambridge University Press.

Norris, M. L., and Cunningham, D. R. (1981). Social impact of hearing loss in the aged. *Journal of Gerontology, 36*, 727-729.

Oyer, E. J. (1976). Exchanging information within the older family. In H. J. Oyer and E. J. Oyer (Eds.), *Aging and communication.* Baltimore: University Park Press.

Oyer, E. J., and Paolucci, B. (1970). Homemakers' hearing losses and family integration. *Journal of Home Economics, 62*, 257-262.

Parenti, M. (1978). *Power and the powerless.* New York: St. Martin's Press.

Posner, J. D. (1982). Particular problems of antibiotic use in the elderly. *Geriatrics, 37*, 49-54.

Powers, J. K., and Powers, E. A. (1978) Hearing problems of elderly persons. *ASHA, 20*, 79-83.

Rodin, J., and Langer, E. J. (1977). Long term effects of a control-relevant intervention with the institutionalized aged. *Journal of Personality and Social Psychology, 35*, 897-902.

Rosenwasser, H. (1964). Otitic problems in the aged. *Geriatrics, 19*, 11-17.

Sadock, B. J., Kaplan, H. I., Freedman, A. M., and Sussman, N. (1975). Psychiatry in the urban setting. In A. M. Freedman, H. I. Kaplan, and B. J. Sadock; (Eds.), *Comprehensive textbook of psychiatry (Vol. II).* Baltimore: Williams & Wilkins.

Schachter, F. F. (1979). *Everyday talk to toddlers: Early intervention.* New York: Academic Press.

Schein, J. D. (1984). Personal communication.

Schlesinger, H. S., and Acree, M. C. (1984). Paper presented at the National Conference on Habilitation and Rehabilitation of Deaf Adolescents, Wagoner, OK.

Schlesinger, H. S., and Meadow, K. P. (1972). *Sound and sign.* Berkeley: University of California Press.

Schow, R. L., Christensen, J. M., Hutchinson, J. M., and Nerbonne, M. A. (1980). *Communication disorders of the aged.* Baltimore: University Park Press.

Schow, R. L., and Nerbonne, M. A. (1982). Communication screening profile: Use with elderly clients. *Ear and Hearing, 3*, 135-147.

Seligman, M. E. (1975). *Helplessness.* San Francisco: W. H. Freeman.

Sherman, S. W., and Robinson, N. M. (Eds.) (1982). *Panel on testing of handicapped people* (Committee on Ability Testing). Washington, DC: National Academy Press.

Singerman, B., Riedner, E., and Folstein, M. (1980). Emotional disturbance in hearing clinic patients. *British Journal of Psychiatry, 137*, 58-62.

Slaughter, D. (1970). Parental potency and the achievements of inner city black children. *American Journal of Orthopsychiatry, 40*, 433-440.

Snow, C. E. (1977). The development of conversation between mothers and babies.

Journal of Child Language, 3, 34-52.

Staff, Institute for Information Studies (1983). The results of helping: Empowerment or helplessness? *Rehab Brief, 6,* 7.

Stahlecker, J. E. (in press). Application of the strange situation attachment paradigm to a neurologically impaired population. *Child Development.*

Suls, J. (1982). Social support, interpersonal relations, and health. In G. S. Sanders and J. Suls (Eds.), *Social psychology of health and illness.* Hillsdale, NJ: Lawrence Erlbaum Associates.

Ventry, I. M., and Weinstein, B. E. (1982). The hearing handicap inventory for the elderly. *Ear and Hearing, 3,* 128-134.

Von der Lieth, L. (1972). Experimental social deafness. *Scandinavian Audiology, 1*(2), 81-87.

World Health Organization (1959). *Mental health problems of aging and the aged.* Geneva: World Health Organization.

Zarit, S. H. (1980). *Aging and mental disorders.* New York: Free Press.

Zetzel, E. R. (1965). Dynamics of the metapsychology of the aging process. In M. A. Berezin and S. H. Cath (Eds.), *Geriatric psychiatry.* New York: International Universities Press.

Zigler, E., and Butterfield, E. C. (1968). Motivational aspects of changes in IQ test performance of culturally deprived nursery school children. *Child Development, 39,* 1-4.

Zigler, E., and Trickett, P. K. (1978). IQ, social competence, and evaluation of early childhood intervention programs. *American Psychologist, 33,* 789-798.

Zimbardo, P. G., Andersen, S. M., and Kabat, L. G. (1981). Induced hearing deficit generates experimental paranoia. *Science, 212,* 1529-1531.

Chapter **8**
Adjustment to Acquired Hearing Loss: A Working Model

James G. Kyle, Lesley G. Jones, and Peter L. Wood

The vast majority of those individuals passing through audiological services have relatively mild hearing losses. Their personal, social, and vocational needs have been anticipated but never effectively dealt with in the United Kingdom and have received very little research attention in any country. The authors are concerned here with these needs and particularly with the individual's adjustment. Our understanding of adjustment is extremely limited and our expectations of those with an acquired hearing loss are poorly defined. We offer a working model of the adjustment process that is currently undergoing analysis. The extent to which this process is understood may determine our success in rehabilitation.

APPROACHING THE PROBLEM

Acquired hearing loss has been something of a Cinderella in social research on deafness. Most research time and money has been spent on those with prelingual deafness, especially children. In addition, acquired hearing loss has been associated with aging and supposed declining capabilities of elderly persons. The few United Kingdom organizations for the "hard-of-hearing" have drawn their members from senior citizens and their practices from long-standing caring attitudes. The population with which we are concerned here lies between those whose loss arises in the early or late stages of life. Without obvious organizational support or social awareness, they have to cope with declining hearing at work, at home, and in social settings. The complexity of their task of adjustment and its effects on others have never been fully appreciated or adequately researched.

Hearing loss is widespread; Leske (1981) has claimed that it is the most common source of disability in the United States. In the United Kingdom, the MRC Institute of Hearing Research (1981) indicates that

Table 8-1.   Percentage of Population with Better-Ear Hearing Loss Above 25 dB and 45 dB, by Age: United Kingdom, 1981

	Percentage above	
Age	*>25 dB*	*>45 dB*
21-30	1	0
31-40	5	1
41-50	10	2
51-60	23	6
61-70	34	17
71 and over	74	49

Adapted from Davis, A. C. (1983). Hearing disorders in the population. In M. E. Lutman and M. P. Haggard (eds.): *Hearing science and hearing disorders*. London: Academic Press.

almost 20 per cent of the population have hearing losses above 25 dB. However, there are marked differences according to age, the proportion with a loss over 25 dB in the better ear rising from 5 per cent among persons 31 to 40 years old to 74 per cent among those over 70 (Table 8-1).

The 5 to 23 per cent of persons between 31 and 60 years of age with a hearing loss of 25 dB or more in the better ear have a severe task coping with family relationships and employment. In addition, this population is less likely than older persons to acquire hearing aids (Davis, in press), and up to a quarter will not seek an audiological test (Haggard, Foster, and Iredale, 1981).

Almost certainly, the process of adjustment begins before the individual is even aware of his or her hearing loss. Hearing problems can arise in situations in which the individual may have reasons for not hearing or is allowed (by asking for repetition) to "re-hear" a missed message. There is very little research on this critical period when hearing loss begins, before an audiological diagnosis is made. Virtually all research on acquired hearing loss deals with the period after services are provided.

One of our interests in this chapter and in our research is to consider why so few people seek help with their hearing loss and how they cope in both personal and social terms. Equally important, of course, is the period after the diagnosis, when the individual can choose to be more open about the loss. We will argue that these constitute two different phases of the adjustment process and have to be treated differently if we are to understand how well an individual eventually copes.

The views of hearing people on the nature of coping are often simple; for example, coping involves the "acceptance" of hearing loss and reduced access to social situations. However, the hearing aid is expected to make sound clear and, if the user can tolerate the initial stages of discomfort, the benefits will become apparent. Ideally, those at home will understand the problems and strike a balance between supportiveness and dominance that will allow the hearing-impaired person to be effective and independent, and to participate in family life.

Unfortunately, this seems rarely to be the case and no United Kingdom service is set up to counsel the family or to deal with the nature of coping. We have only a hazy idea of how to advise an individual to cope and, indeed, the prime target of research on coping has been to estimate and then measure the use of the hearing aid and other services. Few researchers have actually asked those with a hearing loss how they feel they are dealing with their problem. Thomas and Herbst (1980) found the traditional higher incidence of mental ill-health in people with a hearing problem. Loneliness, so often attributed to those with acquired hearing loss (e.g., Bunting, 1981), is also found in such studies (Kyle and Wood, 1983; Thomas and Herbst, 1980). In effect, the evidence points to a lack of "coping" and to inappropriate adjustment, which leads to dissatisfaction. Whether improved counseling would have any effect is arguable, but unless we have some view of what constitutes adequate adjustment, we cannot offer advice about what an adult who loses his hearing should anticipate. We must find an explanatory model of the adjustment process that allows meaningful evaluation of adaptation to hearing loss.

Knapp (1948) suggests that a stable personality prior to the onset of hearing loss is the prime indicator of subsequent adjustment. But our ability to measure adequately the stability of an individual's personality prior to hearing loss onset is, at best, rather limited. When, as in most cases, the onset has been gradual, this task becomes almost impossible. People with an acquired hearing loss arrive for rehabilitation with an unknown, or incompletely verifiable, background. It is also vital to examine the environment in which the individual functions and the people who inhabit it. This has become a major focus of our work, and what we can offer here is a working hypothesis of how deafness occurs in the social and psychological world of the individual. It is only an initial attempt to deal with a very complex problem; we offer it as a model to be critically examined. We will explore the basis of the model and the data which we have collected so far that led us to this view.

A MODEL OF HEARING LOSS AND ADJUSTMENT

Our ideas have arisen from three research projects conducted in Bristol that have successively focused on social and vocational implications, hearing aid use, and adjustment and the family. In each case we have interviewed those with acquired hearing loss, and we are currently interviewing them and their partners at home. What follows is a synthesis of our findings that depicts the development of hearing loss and subsequent adjustment.

Our model is based on the following set of simple ideas:

1. Individuals live and work in information environments governed by social and personal norms as well as access features such as speed, intensity, and density of information.

2. Individuals, through personal and social adjustment, attempt to control the access features of the information they receive.

3. In normal circumstances, most people have adjusted to a specific level of control of these features, which varies from one individual to another but is negotiated and agreed upon in any social circumstances.

4. The onset of hearing loss disturbs the control that the individual can exert.

5. In terms of access, the individual's initial response is to increase the intensity, the repetition, or the concentration level to maximize the information being received.

6. This overt additional control may be unacceptable to others in social situations and produces a realization of "hearing loss."

7. There are at least three solutions: (a) increase the level of control at all costs; (b) accept or expect a reduced level of control and flow of information; and (c) reject or avoid situations in which the level of control is threatened. All three can be adopted by any individual.

8. The degree to which an individual can tolerate the reduced and varying access to information at home and work will determine the degree of adjustment.

Phases in Acquisition of Hearing Loss

To explain our approach, we must consider three phases in the acquisition of hearing loss: first, the period before the individual acknowledges the loss and encounters medical services; second, the diagnosis and referral period; and third, the period after diagnosis and likely hearing aid provision.

Phase 1. The Loss Is Not Acknowledged

Phase 1 may vary from a period of a few days to 20 or 30 years or more. Although conscious realization of hearing impairment may occur relatively late or never, adjustment occurs in every case. This phase corresponds to the time between initial onset and a visit to a doctor or clinic. According to the Medical Research Council (1981), up to 75 *per cent* of those with acquired hearing loss are in this phase at any one time. These are people without hearing aids who have never visited a rehabilitation agency.

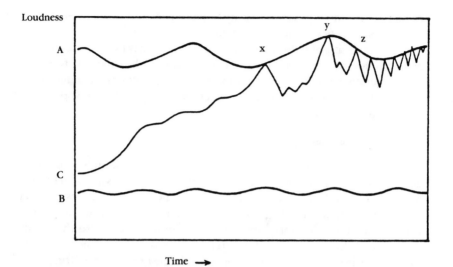

Figure 8-1.   First Phase: Increasingly regular testing of socially acceptable loudness levels

Figure 8-1 offers a view of this phase along a dimension of access most affected by hearing loss—the intensity or loudness of sound. In this situation, *A* represents the varying socially acceptable upper limit of sound information—for example, the level acceptable to make oneself understood will be higher at a football match than at home at mealtimes. *B* represents the level usually negotiated by the individual prior to deafness and the amount of eye contact and degree of attention received. At this level, mishearing can occur without alarm.

C represents the response of an individual to deteriorating hearing, with increased control of loudness and the increased use of social and physical means to enhance the intensity of information. In this phase, the individual tends to increase the volume of television and radio, sit closer to the speaker at meetings, concentrate more when given instructions at work, request louder speech from people on the telephone, and often ask others to repeat. Gradually the frequency of this "adjustment" approaches socially acceptable levels. At points *x*, *y*, *z*, and so on, the levels breach the social norm, and must be immediately reduced because of social pressure. A family member remarks on the television volume, people may put their hands over their ears, and there are refusals to repeat statements ("it doesn't matter"). In each case, the individual realizes he has exceeded a social norm, even though he may not see it as an important one or realize that his control of loudness has contributed to it. The outcome is, nevertheless, a reduced level of loudness or alienation of others (and thereby reduction in control). As the hearing-impaired person approaches referral, these situations occur more frequently.

The realization of the source of this problem may be limited. Doctors and audiologists report that many people go for a hearing test to satisfy family members, not because they think anything is wrong. A denial of the permanence of the loss ("It's only sometimes that I don't hear well") may indicate that adjustment is taking place.

Phase 2: Diagnosis And Prescription

In this period, which generally lasts a few months, the individual must accept the fact that he or she has a permanent hearing loss and will have to wear a hearing aid. This phase consists of the time between the first contact with a professional and diagnosis and the receipt of a hearing aid. In the United Kingdom, the normal procedure is an interview with the family doctor at the local health center, referral to a hospital or audiology clinic for tests, return to the doctor or clinic for the test results and fitting of an aid, and a final visit to receive the aid.

During this period, great uncertainty is experienced. The diagnosis of decreasing hearing presents a wide range of unpleasant prospects: loss of all hearing; loss of job, independence, and control of social situations; rejection by family and friends; and fear of perceived stigma. This period of uncertainty may be counteracted by the adjustment achieved in Phase 1, previous contact with and knowledge of hearing loss, and the coping capacity of the family and social environment. The personal, social, and vocational consequences of hearing loss must be faced. People must be told of the hearing problem; the newly acquired hearing aid provides an opportunity for this, but their responses are uncertain.

Phase 3: Subsequent Accommodation

Most of the literature on acquired hearing loss deals with Phase 3. This is a period when "adjustment" has been expected, but when further hearing loss and increasing withdrawal and the entrenchment of defensive behavior are likely. The initial support of family and friends must be replaced by a long-term commitment. Continued involvement with "disability" can be as difficult for the family as for the individual. Unfortunately, their attitudes are often out of phase. The hearing-impaired person feels that family members do not adequately understand, since they have not experienced the loss nor been aware of it long enough. Family members feel that the individual has become self-centered and has not "accepted" or "adjusted to" his hearing loss.

Inevitably, the struggle to maintain information levels continues. The degree of social and environmental contact will vary with the type of hearing loss and the successful use of the hearing aid. Each person tries to maintain the accustomed level of control of each situation at home, at work, and in society. Unless the aid is very helpful, and we have found few such cases, adjustment processes must deal with diminished control. Two alternatives arise. Behavior can be changed either (1) to increase control (for example, an introvert can become an extrovert to try to dominate interaction) or (2) to withdraw from situations that threaten independence and control. The latter is more likely.

The perceived dependence of the hearing-impaired person is also a problem. When, for instance, the hearing-impaired husband is unwilling to go to a party, he may say he is tired or not interested ("they only gossip, they never talk about anything important"). In fact, he means that the others do not understand what his hearing loss is like. Recognizing that he will miss parts of the conversation and feel left out, his wife offers support and interpretation when necessary. She thinks he has not come to terms with his loss and the need to accept help.

In fact, his need is for self-determination or control, the chance to select the information he wants, to control the conversation at times, and to participate at his accustomed level. Indirect control through his wife's interpretation does not allow the social monitoring he wishes. Hence, his only alternative is to withdraw. If he is forced into the situation, outcomes such as those depicted in Figure 8-2 are likely: a lower level of information flow or repeated breaching of social norms. The result is to increase his future resistance to such "no-win" situations. The reduced control of

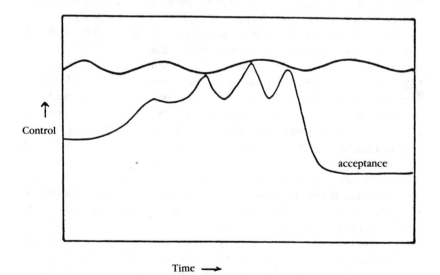

Figure 8-2.   Phase 3: Initial high expectancy of control challenges norms and is replaced by low expectancy

information and the direct attack on his independence merely increase his awareness of his handicap.

The strength of these feelings and reactions will vary with (1) the degree of loss, (2) previous dependence level, (3) the explicitness of family interaction, and (4) the family's tolerance for the changes. One would not expect a crisis or disaster, although marital breakdown and suicide attempts occur. In the vast majority of cases, a level of everyday interaction will be reached which, though not ideal for the hearing-impaired person, constitutes the new lifestyle. The type of job and the type of support from family and friends will determine how frequently social control problems arise (as in Figure 8-2), but these should decrease with time. During Phase 3, the individual reaches a stable mode still character-ized by control problems.

Phases of Adjustment

The situations described are familiar and their interpretation is not necessarily novel or illuminating. However, with this model we can now predict situations and outcomes that can be manipulated to facilitate adjustment. Such predictions can aid the counselor to help the individual to restructure his world to enhance his effectiveness.

Adjustment: Phase 1

The prereferral stage is of considerable importance. Davis (1983) de-scribes the attempts of the National Study of Hearing to determine accurate incidence figures for the United Kingdom. Around 12,000 randomly chosen names from electoral registers were classified using a brief ques-tionnaire, and over 700 persons were then tested at a clinic. The incidence of hearing levels of 35 dB and over in the better ear was estimated at 8 per cent of the population, although only 4 per cent had an aid. About 8 per cent of manual compared to 3 per cent of non-manual workers reported a hearing loss. Since 3 per cent of both groups owned a hearing aid, the greater reluctance of manual workers to accept this free health service is evident.

We would predict this from our model of perceived control. Those with nonmanual jobs are more likely to employ verbal social control, to recognize the effect of their hearing loss, and to obtain a hearing aid. As manual workers have less expectation of personal control, the conflicts depicted in Figure 8-1 are less likely to arise in their work. Accordingly, they are less likely to acquire hearing aids. Bunting's survey (1981) of public attitudes confirms that the workplace is a key area for contact with people with a hearing loss, suggesting that the control issue is much more apparent in this setting.

Early research suggested that personality and stability before hearing loss were crucial in determining the prognosis after hearing loss. However, these studies (Knapp, 1948; Levine, 1960) did not deal adequately with the problem of establishing the time of onset (in other than traumatic loss) or of controlling for the errors in retrospective personality assessments. Determining the age of onset is difficult. Kyle and Wood (1983) found that 58 per cent of those 25 to 55 years old stated that their deafness began gradually, over a period of a year or two; another 24 per cent reported that their deafness occurred over a period of a few months. Phase 1 can typically last a number of years.

Kyle and Wood (1983) dealt only with those who had reached the referral stage, omitting a large group whose Phase 1 was still ongoing. When asked how they had noticed their hearing loss, their respondents replied, "in conversation" (not in situations like watching television or using the telephone). This would fit our model, since in situations when control can not be exercised, that is, when telling people to speak up is socially unacceptable, the awareness of hearing loss rises. In a telephone conversation, one may think "the line is bad" even if the other party can hear clearly, and when watching television one can readily increase the volume.

Bunting's (1981) survey found that 20 per cent of respondents had a "hearing problem but no hearing aid"; the General Household Survey (1977) reported that 14 per cent of a sample of 23,047 people were in the same category. There is an obvious need to study this large group of people in Phase 1 of hearing loss adjustment to understand the full range of hearing loss problems in the population.

Adjustment: Phase 2

In the United Kingdom, Phase 2 is of short duration. Kyle and Wood (1983) report that 51 per cent of those in their study were referred immediately by their family doctor to audiological services; another 42 per cent were referred within a few months. It is in this period that "the coming to terms with hearing loss" must occur. It is not clear how traumatic this situation generally is. Our arguments about Phase 1 imply an increasing acceptance. In Phase 2, rehabilitation counseling should begin, describing the nature of the loss and how it will affect the individual's social and personal life. Unfortunately, in our study we found little evidence of this counseling. Forty-two per cent of respondents said that no explanation of their hearing loss was given by professionals; it was mainly the ear, nose, and throat consultant who offered an explanation (Table 8-2). Few people received advice on personal adjustment.

As shown in a subsequent study (Kyle and Wood, 1984), counseling was centered on the use of the hearing aid. Fifty-five per cent of respond-

Table 8-2.   Explanations of Hearing Loss Given by Professionals

	Percentage* Giving Explanation of:		
Professional	Physical Loss	Effects on Work and Socializing	Effects on Communication
Doctor	15	0	0
Specialist†	55	4	6
Audiologist	5	4	2

* Of 105 respondents with mild to profound, predominantly moderate, hearing loss (Kyle and Wood, 1983; hearing loss functional rating scale based on Schein and Delk, 1974).
    †Ear, nose, and throat consultant.

ents were shown how to clean it, and 87 per cent how to change batteries; 55 per cent were told it would take time to get used to the hearing aid; 42 per cent were told that different situations would require different approaches; 37 per cent were told about the type of sound from the aid; 13 per cent were shown how to use the aid with a telephone; 5 per cent were informed about other appliances such as television adaptors and flashing alarms. Not surprisingly, 89 per cent of respondents reported frustration. At this crucial stage of personal and social adjustment the services concentrate on the appliance, not the individual. There has been little personal counseling. This view is confirmed by a recent collection of papers surveying the field (Watts, 1983).

Many studies by audiologists and physicians have tended to explain the use of hearing aids in terms of their physical performance and appearance, neglecting social and personal factors. Rehabilitation services are considered successful if they follow up after the initial provision of aids and increase their use (Brooks, 1979). Clearly, in the United Kingdom, Phase 2 tends to be dominated by the supplying of hearing aids, and support services are designed to promote hearing aid use. The potential offered by the hearing therapy services in some health districts has not yet been nationally fulfilled.

There is a considerable literature on the effects of general medical diagnosis on personal and family situations (e.g. Thomas, 1978; Hannam, 1977) and extensive case studies (e.g., Booth and Statham, 1982). A general stage model with a degree of currency implies that diagnosis of illness is followed first by shock, anxiety, denial, and disbelief (Burr, Good, and del Vecchio-Good, 1978) and then by guilt, self-blame, depression, and even grief reactions (Cobb, 1976). None of these models has dealt with acquired hearing loss, and our experience indicates far less traumatized responses. However, United Kingdom health care services give no attention to them. Our control model is of limited use, since Phase 2 is characterized by most individuals' passive, consumer orientation to health serv-

Table 8-3.   Concerns Expressed During Diagnosis

Concern	Percentage* expressing	
	Personal concern	*View of family concern*
How I can communicate with others	84	60
How it will affect job	79	50
How it will affect me	76	69
How it will affect family life	74	55
How it will affect social life	71	48

From Kyle, J. G., and Wood, P. (1984). Changing patterns of hearing aid use and level of support. *British Journal of Audiology.* Reprinted with permission.

* Of 38 respondents with mild to severe hearing loss; functional rating scale based on Schein and Delk, 1974.

ices. In effect, adjustment is prescribed in relation to the hearing aid, and hopes for control and independence focus on striving to wear the aid.

People remain concerned about the personal implications of hearing loss, but their concerns now differ from those ascribed to family members (Table 8-3).

Thus, Phase 2 is a period of resolution of doubt, when a diagnosis of hearing loss is made and the prospects of continued and further loss are to be faced. Our investigations provide no indication that United Kingdom health care services are prepared to deal with the great social, psychological, and personal impact of this phase on subsequent adjustment. Not surprisingly only 24 per cent of respondents felt that their hearing aids would be easy or straightforward to use; 53 per cent were embarrassed by their aid in social situations, even when it was a small, behind-the-ear type (Kyle and Wood, 1984).

Hence, the individual's adjustment to hearing loss is almost in abeyance during Phase 2, with a belief that the hearing aid will solve the major problems. Bunting (1981) found that 45 per cent of her random population thought that hearing aids were useful in all situations. Our evidence suggests that this view is shared by hearing-impaired people, who have assumed that a hearing aid can restore their level of control.

Adjustment: Phase 3

Most research on acquired hearing loss has dealt with what happens in Phase 3, the period after a hearing aid has been provided, when adaptation by the individual has to take place.

We thought his hearing aid had broken down so we went to have it checked. They told us there was nothing wrong with it but he would have to come back the following week for a hearing test. At the end, the doctor was going to tell him but I said, "He can't hear you, you'll have to write it down" so he wrote on a piece of paper, "You're deaf." Dan was shocked ... he wrote back "For life?" The doctor wrote back, "Yes" and that was it. We came away stunned ... with nothing.

This dramatic Phase 3 episode (in the words of the wife of a man with a minor loss leading to a Phase 3 start in profound deafness) illustrates the force of simple events. The brief phrases, the writing down, and the emptiness produce a crisis that the family must usually face on their own.

We can divide research on Phase 3 into four main areas: adjustment to hearing aids, personal and social adjustment, vocational adjustment, and family adjustment.

Adjustment to Hearing Aids Rehabilitation services in advanced countries are concerned with hearing aid use. Greater hearing aid use tends to be the goal, but we have found little evidence of extended advice on the situations in which aids can most effectively be used. Studies focus on the amount of hearing aid use and view the hearing-impaired as clients or consumers. Stephens (1977) reviewed post-war studies indicating that a large proportion of those with aids rarely or never used them. The proportion has varied from 41 per cent (Kodicek and Garrad, 1955) to 70 per cent (Brooks, 1972). Miniaturization and extensive rehabilitation services such as those in Denmark (Pedersen, Frankner, and Terkildsen, 1974) greatly increase the use of aids. Brooks (1979, 1981) and Haggard and colleagues (1981) are optimistic about how hearing aid support increases use, although neither provides unequivocal data and both deal with older populations than we are discussing here.

However, Haggard and associates (1981) suggest that most benefit was obtained from the hearing aid when listening to radio and television news and least benefit when someone spoke from another room. The first is a situation of maximal control of sound intensity; the second is a situation of significantly reduced control.

Kyle and Woods' (1984) comparisons of situations when aids were used "within the first two weeks" and "at the present time" indicate a pattern that can be interpreted in terms of control features. Hearing aid use is generally greater at work than at home and use "now" is significantly less than at the beginning of Phase 3. There is some agreement, but no statistically significant relation, between situations in which communication was easy or difficult (Kyle and Wood, 1983) and in which an aid was useful, indicating a complex interaction of factors in communication. In effect, hearing aid performance does not adequately predict communication performance for the people in this study. As we will see in the next section, communication ease tends to follow the prediction of levels of control. The research on hearing aid use does not suggest that it is the single key area for the adjustment of hearing-impaired people. Yet in the United Kingdom it is the primary target of research and service delivery. There is clearly a need to look at other factors in the adaptation of hearing-impaired people.

Personal and Social Adjustment Most personal accounts of acquired hearing loss tend to focus on the traumatic aspects of the loss (e.g. Lehman, 1954; Hunt, 1944). Characteristically, people with acquired loss become anxious, withdrawn, suspicious, hostile, isolated, and lonely (Denmark, 1969). Personality questionnaires provide the stereotype highlighted by Markides and co-workers (1979) of increasing depression, discouragement, suspicion of friends and family, oversensitivity, irritability, and, occasionally, paranoia. The literature suggests that most people who acquire a hearing loss are maladjusted.

Thomas and Herbst (1980) attempted to overcome the methodological and sampling problems characteristic of nearly all previous studies, but still reinforced the finding of loneliness. Despite their tentativeness in presenting their findings, they confirm the stressful nature of hearing loss and its direct effect on self-image.

Social problems have also been extensively attributed to acquired hearing loss. Beethoven wrote in 1802:

> If I appear in company I am overcome by a burning anxiety, a fear that I am running the risk of letting people notice my condition . . . . Such experiences have almost made me despair and I was on the point of putting an end to my life—the only thing which held me back was my art.

Both Levine and Denmark explain these problems as a loss of autonomy in social situations. Breed, van den Horst, and Mous (1980) present a version of this view: the anxiety and loss of autonomy restricts attempts to create new friendships. Most persons in Beattie's (1981) study considered that the quality of their social life had been adversely affected and 60 per cent rated conversation in groups as the most difficult.

As can be seen, most of the literature concerns what is implicitly perceived as maladjustment arising from a disabling condition. It is relatively easy to confirm these findings but rather more problematic to understand aspects of coping or positive strategies that might explain them. Knapp (1948) outlined five, primarily maladjustment, strategies: (1) overcompensation—adopting an extrovert style, with great emphasis on talking to reduce the degree of lipreading required; (2) denial—attempting to lead the same lifestyle as before; (3) retreat from society—withdrawal from social interaction because of its difficulty; (4) somatic complaints—neurotic displacement producing a range of "illnesses"; and (5) exploitation—the adoption of a badge of invalidization to gain sympathy and exploit others.

Table 8-4.   Percentage of Respondents Communicating with Ease in Given Situations*

Situation	Percentage
Home at mealtimes	78
With a doctor	76
Buying gasoline	66
General conversation at home	45
Telephone	35
Neighbor's call	23
Tea break	19
Banks and shops	17
Job interview	17
Buying train tickets	13
Paying bus fare	12
Conversation in street	11
Conversation at bus stop	10
Pubs and restaurants	5

* Percentage of 105 respondents with mild to profound, predominantly moderate, hearing loss finding it easy or very easy to communicate in these situations (Kyle and Wood, 1983).

One can see how these come to be accepted and are built into the negative stereotype of acquired hearing loss. In practice, acquired loss is less traumatic and severe than described in the literature. Here, we adopt a longer perspective: adjustment begins in Phase 1, not Phase 3, and therefore most of these features are working styles that have produced an equilibrium of coping for the individual. They are not merely negative outcomes, even when their effects appear to limit the individual's potential.

Kyle and Wood (1983) asked people about the reality of their response to situations. Table 8-4 shows the pattern of increasing communication difficulty as control passes from the individual to other people. Our model predicts that situations where control cannot be exerted and the communication problem is exposed are those most likely to be avoided. People will avoid face-to-face group situations or those where the initiation of conversation or topic cannot be controlled.

We would therefore qualify all of Knapp's strategies by examining the situations in which they occur and attempting to understand how each strategy constitutes an adjustment from the hearing-impaired person's point of view.

Often, acceptance of deafness is assumed to be a prime goal of rehabilitation counseling. When we asked people how they coped with situations (Kyle and Wood, 1983), virtually everyone rejected the strategy of "telling people about their deafness." In situations like those cited in Table 8-4, no more than 6 per cent adopted the strategy of explaining that they were hearing-impaired. For example, 89 per cent of respondents reported difficulties in street conversations but 79 per cent would not tell people that they had a hearing problem. These results were all the more striking since, during this time, a national "sympathetic hearing scheme" was launched, whereby staff in banks and shops were trained to deal with people who identified themselves as deaf. This denial of hearing loss is rational in terms of preserving a self-image, but dysfunctional from a control point of view and will almost certainly lead to rejection of situations that produce the dilemma.

Further questions tend to confirm that hearing-impaired people hold negative views of themselves. Under our model, positive strategies would increase the access to information in situations where control is assured. Hearing-impaired people therefore read considerably more than is the norm: 97 per cent read books every day or regularly, compared with 60 per cent of hearing people and 17 per cent of prelingually deaf people (Kyle and Wood, 1983); 98 per cent read a newspaper every day; 57 per cent watch television every night, compared with only 22 per cent of hearing and 50 per cent of prelingually deaf people. Information within the control of the individual is maximized and situations where the control is threatened or impossible are avoided.

Clearly, more data are needed on the styles of interaction throughout Phases 1, 2, and 3 to test our analysis and to provide a basis for understanding personal adjustment.

Vocational Adjustment. The primary focus of research has been on change of job as a result of hearing loss; however, only a minority usually change their job. Figures range from 4 per cent (Kyle and Wood, 1983) to 11 per cent (Thomas and Herbst, 1980) to 24 per cent (Beattie, 1981), and even to a massive 50 per cent (Cottin, 1973). There are sampling differences in each study, none completely achieving a random sample of people of employment age. More faith can be had in the generally agreed statement of lower job status and promotion prospects as a result of hearing loss. Kyle and Wood (1983) measured job satisfaction among hearing-impaired people and found that they had greater satisfaction in jobs in which the job characteristics produce less satisfaction in hearing people. Familiarity with a job offers a higher level of control, so that change is not actively sought, as it is by hearing people whose career is still "mobile." Kyle and Wood (1984) report greater use of hearing aids at work than at home; 93 per cent of one group (Kyle and Wood, 1983) reported use of a hearing aid as their communication strategy at work. Our research does not yet tell us much about adjustment at work, though we have found a more positive picture than is often reported.

Jobs with high levels of control, such as professional and management work, offer the possibility of denial as well as overt acceptance. We would expect the adaptation in Phase 1 to serve as a reference for Phase 3 activities, and the acceptable control levels and means of working may be established early in either phase. As we received no more than anecdotes of dysfunction, it seems that more positive, active adjustment emerges at work.

Family Adjustment. Despite general statements of the importance of home support and the effect that hearing loss must have on family members, there has been little actual examination of home and family situations. Breed and coworkers (1980) suggested extra family tensions and reported that children tended to turn increasingly towards the hearing parent. However, we have not found any investigation in which partners and others at home were asked about their responses to the acquired hearing loss.

The literature on deaf children's families and families in crisis because of a key member's illness can help us to predict responses to acquired hearing loss. Shapiro's (1983) review of family reactions to the ill or handicapped child is particularly useful in setting a framework for understanding the family as the basic unit for health care. She suggests that the family system can be described as (1) an open system in continuous interchange with the external world; (2) a complex, intricate organizational structure; (3) a self-regulating, balance system; and (4) a system capable of transformation. "The family system, confronted with continuous internal and external demands for change may be able to respond with growth, flexibility and structural evolution" (p. 914).

In practice, the family tends to deal with problems as a unit and characteristically finds itself in disequilibrium as an initial psychosocial effect of a problem such as diagnosed hearing loss (Goldson, 1981). However, because of the complexity of family relations, it is difficult to predict the outcome of illness or disability. There is little support for the notion that strong family ties, marital solidarity or happiness protect the family against the disruption encountered. Haggerty (1968) suggests that the opposite can occur and that families with disparate ties may be drawn together by the problem.

Research has offered several models of coping. For example, Brickman et al. (1982) proposed four alternatives based on the individual's attribution of responsibility for the problem. Perhaps more relevant to our needs is the (1983) model of control of Shapiro and Shapiro (in press), developed independently from our own. They suggest that control is a fundamental human need. Illness produces vulnerability and coping involves regaining mastery and control, which is linked to the "locus of control." Individuals can exert control to the extent that they see their life as controllable or controlled (i.e., dependent on the acts of others). They then interpret most strategies for coping with illness in the family in terms of active and passive, positive and negative aspects of control. They con-

Table 8-5.   Control Style Interaction and Predictions for Families

Spouse and Family	Hearing-Impaired Person	
	Dominant	*Submissive*
Dominant	Family system at risk	Adjustment occurring
Submissive	Adjustment occurring	Negative features in adjustment

sider denial an active coping strategy, not the negative defense mechanism of psychodynamic theory.

However, we must understand family interaction better to know when counseling intervention can meaningfully occur. We have completed over 90 home interviews in a study of family coping with acquired hearing loss. The hearing-impaired person's style of interaction with others at home, particularly the person's partner, and their compliance or dominance appear to be important. We have encountered very few supposedly classic pictures of rejection or of submission by the hearing-impaired person, and none of the supposed guilt and mourning that models of illness provide. Stability appears to be reached in three of the four possible combinations of control style (Table 8-5).

Table 8-5 is a first approximation: we are only in the preliminary stages of testing these ideas against the complex family responses to hearing impairment. Nevertheless, a more positive, active role must clearly be assigned to the family if we are to understand the adjustment process and enable counseling to work effectively.

IN CONCLUSION

In presenting our brief review of the literature, we have explored alternative ways of examining the adjustment to hearing loss. Previous research has focused on diagnosis and the time immediately thereafter, yet adjustment to acquired hearing loss obviously occurs over a longer period. It is essential that family interaction be understood and employed in counseling. Hitherto, in the United Kingdom, this has not been the practice.

In our attempts to reach random samples of the hearing-impaired population demographically matched with the hearing population at mid-career, it has become clear that the supposed traumatic stages of hearing impairment are relatively uncommon. When they occur, they are devastating and we have much to learn from these situations. Unfortunately, adjustment to traumatic loss is often accompanied by other physical adjustment needs (for example, as a response to an accident in which hearing loss was only part of the damage), and hearing loss may be considered by health care staff and the individual as the lesser problem. In this situation, a medical model prevails whereby treatment precedes cure and hearing loss is expected to be alleviated by careful adjustment. But we cannot then specify what should be done about the hearing loss.

Persons still employed cannot be equated with elderly deaf people as has been done in some studies. The need for control by the former may be much greater, and adjustment at home (with growing children) and at work (with career opportunities) presents different problems. Not surprisingly, given the stress of this period and the general mildness of their hearing loss, this working population has had little involvement with organizations or services for the hearing-impaired. Thomas and Herbst (1980) observed the same lack of involvement in a population with more severe hearing impairment. It is therefore all the more important that the brief and perhaps only contact with support services, at the time of diagnosis and fitting of an aid, be handled correctly.

Rehabilitation and adjustment necessarily involve family and personal factors. This chapter seeks to draw attention to this fact. We hope that additional research and better models can provide a better understanding of adjustment to hearing loss.

REFERENCES

Beattie, J. A. (1981). Social aspects of acquired hearing loss in adults. Unpublished doctoral dissertation, University of Bradford, England.

Beethoven, L. van (1802). *Heiligenstadt document.* Hamburg: Stadtbibliothek.

Booth, T., and Statham, O. J. (1982). *The nature of special education.* London: Croom Helm.

Breed, P. C. M., van den Horst, A. P. J. M., and Mous, T. J. M. (1980). Psychosocial problems in suddenly deafened adolescents and adults. Paper presented at the First International Congress on Hard-of-Hearing, Hamburg.

Brickman, P., Rabinowitz, V. C., Karuza, J. et al. (1982). Models of helping and coping. *American Psychology, 37,* 368-384.

Brooks, D. N. (1972). The use and disuse of Medresco hearing aids. *Sound, 6,* 80-85.

Brooks, D. N. (1979). Counselling and its effect on hearing aid use. *Scandinavian Audiology, 8,* 101-107.

Brooks, D. N. (1981). Use of postaural aids by NHS patients. *British Journal of Audiology, 15,* 79-86.

Bunting, C. (1981). *Public attitudes to deafness.* London: Office of Population Censuses and Surveys.

Burr, B. D., Good, J. B., and del Vecchio-Good, M. (1978). The impact of illness on the family. In R. B. Taylor (Ed.), *Family medicine: Principles and practices.* New York: Springer-Verlag.

Cobb, S. (1976). Social support as a moderator of life stress. *Psychosomatic medicine, 38,* 300-314.

Cottin, R. H. (1973). Consequences sociales et professionelles de l'apparition chez l'adulte d'une surdite profonde ou totale. *Reeducation Orthophonique, 2* (72), 310-332.

Davis, A. C. (1983). Hearing disorders in the population. In M. E. Lutman and M. P. Haggard (Eds.), *Hearing science and hearing disorders.* London: Academic Press.

Davis, A. C. (in press). Epidemiology of hearing disorder. In R. Hinchcliff (Ed.), *Medicine and old age: Hearing and balance.*

Denmark, J. C. (1969). Management of severe deafness in adults. *Proceedings of Royal Society of Medicine, 62,* 965-967.

General Household Survey. (1977). *Survey of households.* London: Office of Population Censuses and Surveys.

Goldson, E. (1981, July-August). The family care centre. *Children Today,* pp. 15-20.

Haggard, M. P., Foster, J. R., and Iredale, F. E. (1981). Use and benefit of post-aural aids in sensory hearing loss. *Scandinavian Audiology, 10,* 45-52.

Haggerty, R. J. (1968). The management of episodic disorders. In M. J. Green and R. J. Haggerty (Eds.), *Ambulatory pediatrics.* Philadelphia: W. B. Saunders.

Hannam, C. (1977). *Parents and mentally handicapped children.* Harmondsworth: Penguin.

Hunt, W. M. (1944, May). Progressive deafness rehabilitation. *Laryngoscope, 54,* 229-234.

Knapp, P. H. (1948). Emotional aspects of hearing loss. *Psychosomatic medicine, 10,* 203-222.

Kodicek, J., and Garrad, J. (1955). The hearing aid in use. *Journal of Laryngology and Otology, 69,* 807-820.

Kyle, J. G., and Wood, P. (1983). *Social and vocational aspects of acquired hearing loss.* Final Report to MSC, School of Education, Bristol.

Kyle, J. G., and Wood, P. (1984). Changing patterns of hearing aid use and level of support. *British Journal of Audiology, 18,* 211-216.

Lehman, R. R. (1954, May). Bilateral sudden deafness. *New York State Journal of Medicine,* 1481-1484.

Levine, E. S. (1960). *The psychology of deafness.* New York: Grune and Stratton.

Leske, M. (1981). Prevalence estimates of communicative disorders in the U.S. *ASHA, 23,* 229-237.

Markides, A., Brooks, D. N., Hart, F. G., and Stevens, F. S. D. G. (1979). Aural rehabilitation of hearing-impaired adults. *British Journal of Audiology, 13,* 7-14.

Medical Research Council Institute of Hearing Research (1981). Population study of hearing disorders in adults. *Journal of Royal Society of Medicine, 74,* 819-827.

Pedersen, B., Frankner, B., and Terkildsen, K. (1974). A prospective study of adult Danish hearing aid users. *Scandinavian Audiology, 3,* 107.

Schein, J. D., and Delk, M. T. (1974). *The deaf population of the United States.* Silver Spring, MD: National Association of the Deaf.

Shapiro, I., and Shapiro, J. (in press). Areas of self control for men and women. *Journal of Clinical Psychology.*

Shapiro, J. (1983). Family reactions and coping strategies in response to the physically ill or handicapped child: A review. *Social Science and Medicine, 17*, 913-931.

Stephens, S. D. G. (1977). Hearing aid use by adults: A survey of surveys. *Clinical Otolaryngology, 2*, 385-402.

Thomas, A. J., and Herbst, K. G. (1980). Social and psychological implications of acquired deafness in adults of employment age. *British Journal of Audiology, 14*, 76-85.

Thomas, D. (1978). *The social psychology of childhood disability*. London: Methuen.

Watts, A. (1983). *Acquired deafness in adults*. London: Croom Helm.

Chapter 9
Adult Hearing Loss and the Family

Herbert J. Oyer and E. Jane Oyer

The family has survived many cultural and social changes and internal crises. It is a durable institution.

Etzioni (1977) has been less optimistic, suggesting that, if the present divorce rate continues to accelerate, not one intact American family will be left by the mid-1990s. However, family scholars have broadened their conceptions of the family to include other configurations and lifestyles than the traditional mother, father, and 1.8 children. Although, as Broderick (1979) observes, over 93 per cent of Americans marry and remarriage rates are also high, nonetheless family forms also include the previously married single female or male parent and the never-married single biological or adopting parent.

Regardless of the family form of the hearing-impaired individual, hearing loss brings certain penalties. Conventional wisdom suggests that the extent of the disruption in normal life-cycle activities is a function of a number of variables including the age at which the loss occurs, the type and magnitude of loss, and the individual's psychological integrity and intellectual capacities. An additional variable of tremendous import is the extent to which family members and friends understand the psychological, social, educational, and vocational implications of hearing impairment and are motivated to initiate and to respond meaningfully to a course of action to support the hearing-impaired person.

At whatever age the loss occurs, its effects on the human communication process is of central concern. In children, educational and social development and feelings of self-worth, which are so dependent upon successful dyadic and small group interaction, are of immediate concern. In adults, the maintenance of successful social relationships in the family and other groups, self-image, and successful performance in the workplace are paramount.

In adults, the principal focus of professional attention has been on (1) measurement of hearing function; (2) the application and use of amplification; and (3) short-term hearing aid orientation, counseling, and rehabilitation (Alpiner, 1978; Davis and Hardick, 1981; Giolas, 1982; Henoch, 1979; Oyer and Frankmann, 1975). Data abound in the first two areas, but are less plentiful in the third (Oyer, 1976; Oyer, 1982). So far as we know, there is virtually no empirical basis for generalizations about the impact of hearing handicap on family and friends. One notable exception is a study of the relationships of homemakers' hearing losses and family integration (Oyer and Paolucci, 1970).

Accordingly, the principal purpose of this paper is to present a model of the effects of hearing loss on family communication from which inferences can be made about the effects upon family relationships. Hopefully, the questions which emerge will indicate the areas in which research is needed as well as some practical rehabilitative measures.

To clarify the importance of hearing loss in adulthood and its implications for relationships in the family, particularly, the older family, we will discuss (1) theoretical approaches to the study of the family, (2) family relationships in later adulthood, (3) the prevalence of hearing loss in late adulthood, (4) the impact of hearing loss in adulthood on the family, (5) a model of hearing impairment and family relationships, and (6) research recommendations and practical suggestions.

THEORETICAL APPROACHES IN FAMILY RESEARCH

The Developmental Approach

Hill and Duvall are generally credited with devising the truly eclectic developmental approach in 1947. Hill and Mattessich (1977, p. 1) state:

> Family development as a theoretical perspective is distinctive among the half dozen recognized conceptual frameworks for family study since it is the only one to have been formulated at the beginning with the conceptual demands of family research and service in the forefront of concern. For example, no other framework attends to the issue of family time, the developments and changes which occur in families over the life span. The scholars who have worked on this framework have unashamedly borrowed and incorporated concepts from a variety of disciplines paying less attention to issues of theoretical elegance than to substantive relevance.

Although the framework was proposed before it was empirically tested, its use of existing concepts gave it a certain immediate credibility. The importance of the family's longitudinal career and changes in family interaction patterns had been recognized.

Some of the differences of opinion about the family life cycle have reflected the system of partitioning used by various researchers. In the five editions of her book, Duvall (1957, 1977) used an eight-stage schema;

Rogers (1964), on the other hand, used a 24-stage plan. Others have made further modifications, but the eight-stage cycle seems to have held up as well as any.

Early contributions of Havighurst, with whom Duvall worked at the University of Chicago, were published in book form in 1948. His notions about individual tasks as growth imperatives were elaborated by Duvall and Hill (1948) to include family developmental tasks. They postulated that individuals meeting their own tasks were also contributing to the fulfill-ment of family developmental tasks—and at some points the two tasks might conflict. The sequential notion that completing the tasks at each stage was essential for a successful transition to the next stage was another key idea. For example, if a young couple did not establish satisfactory intellectual and emotional communication at the outset, they would be expected to have difficulty doing so subsequently.

Erikson (1950) specified that the major task of the adulthood stage could be met either by self-absorption or by generativity (an interest in generations to follow). The major task of the senescent stage would be met with integrity or disgust. Erikson also used an eight-stage typology.

One major advantage of this approach is its focus upon the process of change in the family's development. Rather than portraying a "still shot" of family life, it provided the conceptual tools for a "motion picture." As Hanson (1983, p. 323) states, "the family life cycle is a dynamic concept, capturing the changes that take place in families over time . . . ." Another advantage is that the researcher can examine the family's internal function-ing without excluding its interaction with other social institutions. The developmental approach also offers useful ideas to family life educators and counselors.

In this approach, the oldest child's age is sometimes used as the criterion, indicator, or "readiness period" for movement from one stage to the next. This criterion lacks validity for many modern-day families. A true longitudinal study of the family poses problems for the researcher who may not live long enough to complete it, unless he employs a cross-sectional sample, a retrospective history-taking technique with an elderly group, or several generations of the same family.

Investigating residential preferences and moving behavior over the life cycle, McAuley and Nutty (1982) used a seven-stage plan in their design. Anderson, Russell, and Schumm (1983) used a five-stage scheme in exam-ining perceived marital quality across life-cycle categories.

Hanson (1983) studied individual, family, and historical dimensions of the socioeconomic attainment of working women with a life-cycle approach. Patterson and McCubbin (1983) examined the impact of family life events and changes upon the health of a chronically ill child. McCubbin and Patterson (1983) noted that cystic fibrosis children were affected by certain changes that other family members experienced. The concept of "wholeness"—that each family member is affected by the conduct of every other member—is an integral part of the developmental approach. McCubbin and Patterson (1983) emphasized that families are frequently adjusting simultaneously to multiple life changes.

Reviewing research findings on the impact of an autistic child upon the family at various stages of the life cycle, Harris (1984) observed that the child's presence may intensify the resolution of the conflicts which often accompany the transition between two stages. Can the transition be delayed or movement sometimes arrested—and might this occur in families with a hearing-impaired member?

These researchers who studied the family with the same conceptual approach provided the bases for research questions about the effects of hearing loss on the family. How does hearing loss impinge upon the developmental tasks associated with each stage of family life? How do the effects during the adult stages differ from those in childhood?

A Crisis-Oriented Approach to Family Study

This fascinating approach has enjoyed a fairly long life and has much to recommend it. Although Hanson and Johnson (1979) would like to see some of the concepts changed, their creative alternatives await testing.

The antecedents for this theory (or partial theory) go back at least to the 1930's, but Hill (1949) utilized the approach in his classic work on families undergoing war separations and reunions. His definitions and explications continue to guide researchers (Hanson and Hill, 1964; Hill, 1958; Patterson and McCubbin, 1983). Hill defined a "stressor" as a situation for which a family has had little or no preparation so that members' ability to deal with it is problematic. Stress ensues. A crisis is an event for which normal behavior is inadequate. The resources for meeting a crisis are the strengths (such as goal agreement, communication patterns, and level of education) a family can muster to cope with the stress.

Hill has proposed an *ABCX model*: *A* is the stressor that interacts with *B*, the family's crisis-meeting resources, to produce *C*, the family's definition of the stressor (which determines whether the event becomes a crisis). This chain of reactions culminates in *X*—the crisis. Again, wholeness is a key idea of the system. When a family's equilibrium is disturbed, it will try to reestablish it through the use of the resources available to it. Some believe that the new equilibrium will be the same or lower than before the crisis; others, that the family can learn from such experiences and may achieve a better equilibrium.

Patterson and McCubbin (1983) have added a *pile-up* concept (see also McCubbin and Patterson, 1983). According to this concept, a family can undergo an accumulation of life changes (stressors) simultaneously, which can tax its crisis-meeting resources. The idea is reminiscent of the strains that families and individual members may undergo when trying to meet certain developmental tasks at the same time. Kastenbaum (1979) used a related idea in studies of "grief-depletion" or "grief-overload" reactions to bereavement.

As noted, Patterson and McCubbin (1983) studied the impact that the care of children with chronic cystic fibrosis had on the family. Integrating a modified version of Hill's crisis theory with developmental theory, they examined the relationship between the resulting stress and the child's physical health. Findings indicated that the stress (magnitude of life change) contributed to a decline in physical health. Also, the higher the father's educational level, the better the child's health tended to be. These findings invite fascinating hypotheses about the levels of family functioning and hearing loss (a stressor) at various stages of the life cycle.

FAMILY RELATIONSHIPS IN LATER ADULTHOOD

The steady increase in the number of older people during this century has had far-reaching implications for the family. People born in the United States in 1980 could expect to live nearly 80 years, whereas in 1900 life expectancy was 47 years (Quadagno, 1981). At present, about 26 million people, or 11.5 per cent of the population, are age 65 or older. By the year 2030, 43 million, or 15 to 20 per cent of the population, will be 65 or older (Golanty and Harris, 1982).

The older family reflects the aging population in a number of ways. Whereas, at the turn of the century, most people could not expect to live to old age, now the period after the last child leaves home is far longer than that from marriage through child rearing.

In 1910 the average couple had 4.5 children (Troll, Miller, and Atchley, 1979); today, about 1.8. As family size has decreased, the number of generations living at any one time has increased. Four fifths of older people have living children (Butler and Lewis, 1982). The isolated older family is a myth; most children do not abandon their elderly parents. Four of five older parents see an adult child once a week, and usually more often (Shanas, 1980). Even when distance prevents such visits, ties are generally maintained by phone calls and letters, which Sussman (1976) calls the "modified extended" family. Leigh (1982) found that adults did not disengage from relatives or decrease their interaction with age. With siblings, an hourglass effect was observed. They interacted frequently as children, associated less when rearing their own families, and renewed relationships in their older years. Kinship interaction was normally based upon choice rather than expectation.

According to Quinn (1983), health and the quality of their relationship were the strongest predictors of the psychological well-being of older
parents. Affection and communication were positive influences upon quality. Oyer (1976) noted that several variables, including attitudes, values,
agreement, health-related factors, and the division of labor, may facilitate or
deter communication in the older family. How, then, does an older parent's
severe hearing loss, which impedes easy oral communication, affect her or
his relationship with children and other family members?

Older people are often involved in exchanges of aid with their children, with or without residential propinquity (Lee and Ellithorpe, 1982).
Much aid flows from the older generation to the younger, although it
receives little attention in popular articles on the older family.

As the number of frail elderly persons grows, more middle-aged
daughters are working and have less free time to help their parents (Brody,
1978). Who, then, is going to help them? Johnson and Catalano (1981)
found that nephews and nieces who helped childless uncles and aunts did
so out of loyalty to their parents, not affection for their relatives; the
relationship was not usually intimate and conflicts often arose. Other help
came from siblings and, of course, the spouse. One wonders if families with
a deafened adult exhibit similar helping relationships.

Johnson and Catalano (1983) found that caregivers, usually children
of the "high needs" elderly, may seek to decrease direct support when
needs persist over a long period. However, they played a major role in
helping the dependent elderly to avoid institutionalization. The need for
additional support of families with dependent older parents may be in-
ferred from a report distributed at the recent White House Conference on
Aging (1981, p. 34), which stated, "Although the provision of care by
families to impaired members is extensive, such care may produce serious
negative consequences to the individuals involved of whatever generation." We may speculate about which aspects of family functioning can be
affected by the stressor of hearing loss in the older family.

Early research suggested a low level of happiness or satisfaction in
marital relations in the later years; some termed it the "disenchantment
period." More recent studies, however, have found that most older people
are happy and satisfied with their marriage (Glenn, 1975; Harkins, 1978;
Troll, 1971). Increased companionship and emotional satisfaction have
been rated highly, as in the honeymoon stage; Anderson and colleagues
(1983) found that perceived marital quality does indeed follow a U-shaped
curve. Of course, divorce, desertion, or separation have removed many
unhappy couples from this cohort. Husbands seem to become more nurtur-
ant and wives more instrumental or business-like in their marital roles.

By this time, children have been launched and husbands have been more closely integrated in households. The companionship and interdependence that develop create satisfying relationships but also make loss of a spouse a very difficult adjustment for many survivors. A confidant seems to be an important component of happiness or life satisfaction, because communication plays a critical role in marital and other significant relationships. Again, how does hearing loss affect marital quality during the early, middle, and later stages of the family life cycle?

PREVALENCE OF HEARING LOSS IN LATER ADULTHOOD

Estimates of the prevalence of hearing loss in the population have been derived from National Health Surveys, hearing testing at fairs and other mass gatherings, and individual calculations. Data gathered in the 1962-1963 National Health Survey showed that hearing loss in both ears rose from 3.5 per 1,000 persons under age 17 to 133.0 per 1,000 persons over age 64. Four fifths of those over 44 years of age had some bilateral loss (Oyer, Kapur, and Deal, 1976).

In hearing surveys at three Ohio county fairs, O'Neill (1956) showed that 84.8 per cent of those ages 6 to 9 passed compared to 59.0 per cent of those ages 30 to 39, 12.8 per cent of those 60 to 69 years of age, and none of those age 70 and older. His screening levels were 15 dB at 250, 500, 1000, 2000, 4000, and 8000 Hz. Steinberg, Montgomery, and Gardner (1940) and Webster, Humes, and Lichtenstein (1950) had conducted similar surveys of larger numbers of people.

Rupp (1970) compiled National Health data to show a picture of the increase of hearing impairment with age. At 500, 1000, and 2000 Hz, he found that the rate per 1,000 population rose from 7.9 for persons under 25 years of age to 52.2 for those ages 25 to 64, 129.2 for those 65 to 74 years of age, and 256.4 among those age 75 and over.

Men sustain greater change in auditory sensitivity over time than do women, as shown by eight hearing-level studies from four countries (Davis and Silverman, 1970). The most marked decrement in pure tone sensitivity occurs at high frequencies at age 60 and over for both sexes.

According to Health Interview Survey data (Harris, 1978), auditory problems were second only to arthritis among prevalent selected chronic conditions per 1,000 persons. Close scrutiny of those data showed 33.8 per cent of males age 65 and over with hearing problems, compared with 28.7 per cent with arthritis. Only 26.2 per cent of females in the same age range have a hearing loss but 45.0 per cent have arthritis. As more women join the work force, perhaps hearing loss induced by noise in the workplace will serve to equalize the rate of hearing loss in the two sexes.

IMPACT OF ADULT HEARING LOSS
ON FAMILY AND FRIENDS

Whenever a handicap or abnormal situation hampers communication in a group, a degree of misunderstanding and discomfort can arise.

Surveying elderly persons living in planned housing, Stephens and Bernstein (1984) observed that those with sensory impairments had significantly fewer relationships with family members and other residents. The sensory-impaired and those with chronic and long-term health problems were more socially isolated.

Singer and Brownell (1984) found that older adults knew significantly less about hearing health than did younger adults. If, as Whitelaw and Oyer (1985) found, such knowledge serves to shape attitudes to hearing problems, one might infer that the attitudes could be improved by education and counseling.

Thomas and coworkers (1983) found that elderly hearing-impaired persons were angry and frustrated at having their impairment equated with a decreased ability to function. As Granick, Cleban, and Weiss (1976) and Ohta, Carling, and Harmon (1981) have shown, many people associate hearing loss with reduced mental function.

Hearing-impaired adults tend not to be interested in aural rehabilitation programs. A lack of information and motivation explained why over half of hearing-impaired adults sampled in six clinical settings across the country did not participate in such programs (Oyer et al., 1976). The age range of respondents was 23 to 89 years; those who ignored the recommendation to return for aural rehabilitation, after testing and perhaps hearing aid fitting, were retired or approaching retirement. Thus it appears that it is not a matter of services being unavailable but rather that the adult, particularly the older adult, does not utilize them. This has implications for hearing impairment and family relationships, especially since spouses and friends are included in many rehabilitation programs.

The willingness of adults to acknowledge a hearing loss is another factor affecting family relationships. McDavis (1983-1984) suggests that there is a discrepancy between the amount of loss and the extent of denial: the greatest denial occurs in the range of moderate impairment.

Oyer and Oyer (1979) suggest 14 social consequences of hearing loss for the elderly, all of which may damage family functioning. These include embarrassment associated with failure to understand spoken messages, fatigue from straining to hear, increased irritability and tension, social avoidance and withdrawal, and increased danger from not hearing signals that would alert others. Boredom, rejection, negativism, and depression can have devastating effects on family relationships, as can vulnerability to promises of restored hearing. Reduced information, acting upon misinformation, and reduced leadership opportunities can also have far-reaching effects on the family.

Oyer and Paolucci (1970) showed that the hearing losses of homemakers have significant effects on family relationships. The husbands of women with severe hearing losses had significantly more marital tension, as measured by the Marital Tension Scale of Schaeffer and Bell (1958), than did the husbands of wives with normal hearing. Hard-of-hearing mothers received significantly more help in household tasks from other family members than did mothers with normal hearing. Mothers with hearing loss also spent less time in social activities outside the home. Normal hearing mothers belonged to two organizations and attended 2.5 meetings per month, compared to one organization and one meeting a month for hearing-impaired mothers. Homemakers with normal hearing attached a higher priority to the home as a place to entertain friends, whereas those with hearing loss attached a higher priority to the home as a place for family members. Although the differences were not significant, the hearing-impaired homemakers tended to exercise more power in decision making.

Despite the dearth of such scientific studies on the impact of hearing loss on family relationships, clinicians have abundant case history material on hearing-impaired adults. We know a prominent scientist with impaired hearing who agreed to give a far larger donation than he would have had he not misunderstood the amount requested by a reputable charity in a telephone call. To save face, he donated the funds and ruptured the family budget for months. A sociable and stable middle-aged couple lost virtually all of their close friends because of the wife's unwillingness to acknowledge her hearing loss and seek rehabilitative assistance. Misunderstandings, awkward social situations, and a denial of the loss set them apart and eventually led to a divorce. The reader can doubtless cite other examples of the profound effects that hearing loss can have on family relationships.

A notable account of adventitious deafness in an adult is that of Jack Ashley (1973), the British Member of Parliament. Ashley describes the anger, fear, and frustration that accompanied his loss of hearing and his struggle to remain in Parliament and to sustain his family. In recent statements, Jack and Pauline Ashley (see Chapters 4 and 5) discuss the personal and family ramifications of adventitious deafness and show how the threat to their family was forestalled by insightful and cooperative measures.

Thus, in exploring the impact of hearing loss in adulthood on the family, systematic study, informal observation, and biographical and autobiographical accounts can offer useful approaches. A broader, planned utilization of each approach is needed to provide firm data for generalizations about the impact of adventitious deafness. These could provide a foundation for the development of strategies to help the family meet the crisis of adventitious deafness in adulthood.

A THEORETICAL MODEL OF HEARING IMPAIRMENT AND FAMILY RELATIONSHIPS

Figure 9-1 is a schematic representation of several complex variables in the processes by which hearing loss in adults affects the family. In this theoretical model, we will discuss (1) family life cycle stages, (2) individual and family developmental tasks, (3) stressors, (4) individual and family resources, and (5) levels of family functioning.

Family Life Cycle Stages. As noted earlier, the family life cycle has been partitioned into various numbers of stages, but no one system is *the* best. A grosser typology such as expansion and contraction might be suitable for some studies. A four-stage cycle seemed appropriate for our model, although additional stages—Duvall (1977) suggested eight—can be defended.

Developmental Tasks. Developmental tasks are growth imperatives in each stage of the individual or family life cycle. These competencies are acquired as people work, learn, observe, and proceed to further complexity and mastery. Some tasks are unique to stages such as retirement, but most remain important throughout many stages, although their relative importance may vary. For example, maintaining a home will be a new task for many persons, but a matter of routine to others.

Marrying, communicating, finding compatible friends and becoming intimate with some, and managing time and money are among the tasks that most of us master (Erikson, 1950; Duvall, 1977; Havighurst, 1957). Many of these tasks must also be accomplished by the family as a group: maintaining a meaningful system of communication, socializing with family members, managing resources, and balancing time and energy between family and nonfamily members.

Resources. The means that families employ to reach their goals include resources such as community facilities, individual wealth, energy, time, interests, knowledge, attitudes, and abilities.

Stressor. In this model, the stressor is the hearing impairment of an adult that affects family relationships. Several attempts have been made to assess social adequacy, hearing handicap, and communication function—for example, the Social Adequacy Index of Davis (1948), the self-report of High, Fairbanks, and Glorig (1964), and the communication function of Alpiner, Chevrette, Glascoe, Metz, and Olsen (1974). These are all helpful, although inadequate for determining the impact of hearing loss on family functioning. For our purpose, the instrument should measure the level of individual and family functioning following utilization of individual and family coping resources.

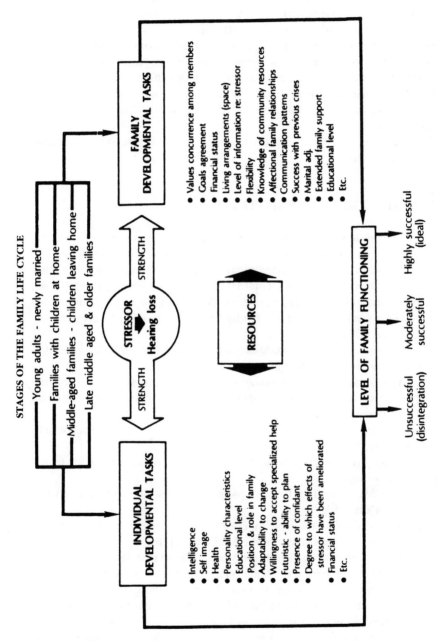

Figure 9-1. Hearing loss and family functioning.

Level of Family Functioning. The level of family functioning in our model depends upon the success with which individual and family resources are utilized in coping with hearing loss. If the resources have been used well, the family will function well. The degree to which individual and family developmental tasks can be successfully accomplished will be determined by the impact of the stressor (hearing impairment) and by the skillful use of coping resources. To quantify the effects of hearing loss on family functioning, it is necessary to quantify the stressor, individual and family developmental tasks, coping resources, and the level of family functioning.

Our model leads to the following suggestions for research and rehabilitative measures.

RESEARCH RECOMMENDATIONS

1. Determine and quantify the factors that comprise each variable in the model: (a) stressor strength—for example, pure tone average, speech reception threshold, discrimination scores, handicap score values; (b) individual developmental tasks; (c) family developmental tasks; (d) individual coping resources; (e) family coping resources; (f) stages (indicators) of the family life cycle; and (g) levels of family functioning.
2. Design and conduct a study to test the model, with suitable methodology and instrumentation.
3. In systematic depth interviews with a national sample of hearing-impaired adults, collect information on the effects of their losses on their development and family functioning.
4. Determine the life-cycle stage(s) at which the family is better able to cope with the stressor.
5. Assess stressor strength in relation to the consequences for family functioning.
6. Identify the family relationships that are most likely to suffer from a parent's hearing loss.
7. Determine how resources for counteracting the effects of hearing loss change at various stages of the family life cycle.
8. Identify the individual and family resources that most effectively combat the deterioration of family relationships due to hearing loss.
9. With hearing loss as the stressor, determine the extent to which the successful completion of individual development tasks predicts the successful completion of family tasks.
10. Determine the extent to which the time and adequacy of aural rehabil-

itation contribute to successful family relationships.

11. Determine the nature and scope of education and counseling that should be provided to hearing-impaired adults, spouses, and family members.
12. Determine the extent to which family relationships vary according to the sex of the person with impaired hearing.
13. Explore the integrative effects that hearing handicap may have on family relationships.

PRACTICAL SUGGESTIONS

1. With the cooperation of hearing-impaired adults, sponsor conferences throughout the country for the education of hearing-impaired adults, relatives, and friends.
2. Provide in-service training on hearing, hearing loss, and the consequences of hearing impairment for the family to health-care givers in homes for the elderly, community centers, and similar settings.
3. Provide courses for allied health and teacher education students about hearing loss in adults and the consequences for families.
4. Hold a small national conference on hearing loss and the family for family counselors and physicians, with regional, state, and local conferences.
5. Offer counseling and education on hearing loss and the family at senior citizen centers.
6. Increase the attention given to adult hearing loss and the family in the mass media.
7. Promote the use and improvement of assistive listening devices in churches, theaters, and other public meeting halls.
8. Urge public and private agencies to support research on adult hearing loss and the family and the development of model formats and procedures for counseling hearing-impaired adults and their families and friends.

REFERENCES

Alpiner, J. G. (1978). (Ed.). *Handbook of adult rehabilitative audiology*. Baltimore: Williams & Wilkins.

Alpiner, J. G., Chevrette, W., Glascoe, G., Metz, M., and Olsen, B. (1971). The Denver Scale of Communication Function. Unpublished, University of Denver.

Anderson, S. A., Russell, C. S., and Schumm, W. R. (1983). Perceived marital quality and family life cycle categories: A further analysis. *Journal of Marriage and the Family, 45*, 1, 127-139.

Ashley, J. (1973) *Journey into silence*. London: The Bodley Head.

Broderick, C. B. (1979). *Marriage and the family.* Englewood Cliffs, NJ: Prentice-Hall.

Brody, E. M. (1978, July). The aging of the family. *Annals of the American Academy of Political and Social Science,* 13-27.

Butler, R. N., and Lewis, M. L. (1982). *Aging and mental health* (3rd ed.). St. Louis: C. V. Mosby.

Davis, H. (1948). The articulation area and the social adequacy index for hearing. *Laryngoscope, 58,* 761-778.

Davis, H., and Silverman, S. R. (Eds.). (1970). *Hearing and Deafness* (pp. 112-113). New York: Holt, Rinehart and Winston.

Davis, J. M., and Hardick, E. J. (1981). *Rehabilitative audiology for children and adults.* New York: John Wiley and Sons.

Duvall, E. M., and Hill, R. L. (1948). *Report of the committee on dynamics of family interaction.* National Conference on Family Life. Washington, D.C.

Duvall, E. M. (1957). *Family development.* Philadelphia: J. B. Lippincott.

Duvall, E. M. (1977). *Marriage and family development.* Philadelphia: J. B. Lippincott.

Erikson, E. H. (1950). *Childhood and society.* New York: Norton.

Etzioni, A. (1977). The family: Is it obsolete? *Journal of Current Social Issues, 14,* 4.

Giolas, T. G. (1982). *Hearing handicapped adults.* Englewood Cliffs, NJ: Prentice-Hall.

Glenn, N. (1975). Psychological well-being in the postparental stage. *Journal of Marriage and the Family, 37,* 105-110.

Golanty, E., and Harris, B. B. (1982). *Marriage and family life.* Boston: Houghton Mifflin.

Granick, S., Cleban, M. H., and Weiss, A. D. (1976). Relationships between hearing loss and cognition in normally hearing aged persons. *Journal of Gerontology, 31,* 434-440.

Hanson, D. A., and Hill, R. (1964). Families under stress. In H. T. Christiansen (Ed.), *Handbook of marriage and the family* (pp. 782-819). Chicago: Rand-McNally.

Hanson, D. A., and Johnson, V. A. (1979). Rethinking family stress theory: Definitional aspects. In W. R. Burr, R. Hill, F. I. Nye, and I. L. Reiss (Eds.), *Contemporary theories about the family* (Vol. 1, pp. 582-603). New York: Free Press.

Hanson, S. J. (1983). A family life-cycle approach to the socio-economic attainment of working women. *Journal of Marriage and the Family, 45*(2), 323-338.

Harkins, E. B. (1978). Effects of empty nest transition on self-report of psychological and physical well-being. *Journal of Marriage and the Family, 40*(3), 544-555.

Harris, C. S. (1978). *Fact book on aging* (p. 110). The National Council on Aging.

Harris, S. L. (1984). The family and the autistic child: A behavioral perspective. *Family Relations, 33*(1), 127-134.

Havighurst, R. J. (1948). *Developmental tasks and education.* University of Chicago Press.

Henoch, M. A. (1979). *Aural rehabilitation for the elderly.* New York: Grune and Stratton.

High, W. S., Fairbanks, G., and Glorig, A. (1964). Scale for self-assessment of hearing handicap. *Journal of Speech and Hearing Disorders, 29,* 215-230.

Hill, R. (1949). *Families under stress.* Westport, CT: Greenwood Press.

Hill, R. (1958). Generic features of families under stress. *Social Casework, 39,* 139-150.

Hill, R., and Mattessich, P. (1977). Reconstruction of family theories: A progress report. Paper presented at the National Council on Family Relations Workshop on Theory Development, San Diego.

Johnson, C. L., and Catalano, D. J. (1981). Childless elderly and their family supports. *Gerontologist, 21*(6), 610-618.

Johnson, C. L., and Catalano, D. J. (1983). A longitudinal study of family supports to impaired elderly. *Gerontologist, 23*(6), 612-618.

Kastenbaum, R. (1979). *Humans developing: A lifespan perspective.* Boston: Allyn and Bacon.

Lee, G. R., and Ellithorpe, E. (1982). Intergenerational exchange and subjective well-being among the elderly. *Journal of Marriage and the Family, 44*(1), 217-224.

Leigh, G. K. (1982). Kinship interaction over the family life span. *Journal of Marriage and the Family, 44*(4), 197-208.

McAuley, W. J., and Nutty, C. L. (1981). Residential preferences and moving behavior: A family life-cycle analysis. *Journal of Marriage and the Family, 44*(2), 301-309.

McCubbin, H., and Patterson, J. (1983). Family stress and adaptation to crisis: A double ABCX model of family behavior. In H. McCubbin, M. Sussman, and J. Patterson (Eds.), *Advances and developments in family stress theory and research* (Vol. 1). New York: Hawarth.

McDavis, K. C. (1983-1984). The effects of severity of hearing impairment and locus of control on the denial of hearing impairment of the aged. *International Journal of Aging and Human Development, 18*(84), 47-59.

Ohta, R. J., Carling, M. F., and Harmon, B. M. (1981). Auditory acuity and performance on the mental status questionnaire in the elderly. *Journal of the American Geriatrics Society, 29*, 476-478.

O'Neill, J. J. (1956). Ohio County Fair Hearing Survey. *Journal of Speech and Hearing Disorders, 21*, 188-197.

Oyer, E. J. (1976). Exchanging information within the older family. In H. J. Oyer and E. J. Oyer (Eds.), *Aging and communication* (pp. 43-61). Baltimore: University Park Press.

Oyer, E. J., and Paolucci, B. (1970). Homemakers' hearing losses and family integration. *Journal of Home Economics, 62*, 257-262.

Oyer, H. J. (1982) Audiological rehabilitation: Research and scholarly efforts 1972-1981. *Journal of Rehabilitative Audiology, 15*, 116-130.

Oyer, H. J., and Frankmann, J. P. (1975). *The aural rehabilitation process.* New York: Holt, Rinehart and Winston.

Oyer, H. J., Freeman, B., Hardick, E., Dixon, J., Donnelly, K., Goldstein, D., Lloyd, L., and Musson, E. (1976). Unheeded recommendations for aural rehabilitation: Analysis of a survey. *Journal of the Academy of Rehabilitative Audiology, 9*, 20-30.

Oyer, H. J., Kapur, Y. P., and Deal, L. V. (1976). Hearing disorders in the aging: Effects upon communication (pp. 175-186). In H. J. Oyer and E. J. Oyer (Eds.), *Aging and communication.* Baltimore: University Park Press.

Oyer, H. J., and Oyer, E. J. (1979). Social consequences of hearing loss for the elderly. *Allied Health and Behavioral Sciences, 2*, 123-138.

Patterson, J. M., and McCubbin, H. I. (1983). The impact of family life events and changes on the health of a chronically ill child. *Family Relations, 32*(2) 255-264.

Quadagno, J. S. (1981). Who are the elderly? A demographic inquiry. In F. J. Berghorn et al. (Eds.), *The dynamics of aging* (pp. 133-149). Boulder, CO:

Westview Press.

Quinn, W. H. (1983). Personal and family adjustment in later life. *Journal of Marriage and the Family, 45*(1), 57-73.

Rogers, R. H. (1964, August). Toward a theory of family development. *Journal of Marriage and the Family*, 262-270.

Rupp, R. R. (1970). Understanding the problems of presbycusis. *Geriatrics, 25*, 100-107.

Schaeffer, E. S., and Bell, R. Q. (1958). Development of a parental attitude research instrument. *Child Development, 29*(3), 339-361.

Shanas, E. (1980). Older people and their families: The new pioneers. *Journal of Marriage and the Family, 42*(1), 9-15.

Singer, J. M., and Brownell, W. W. (1984). Assessment of hearing health knowledge. *The Gerontologist, 24*, 160-166.

Steinberg, J. C., Montgomery, H. C., and Gardner, M. B. (1940). Results of the World's Fair hearing tests. *Journal of Acoustical Society of America, 12*, 291-301.

Stephens, M. A. P., and Bernstein, M. D. (1984). Social support and well-being among residents of planned housing. *The Gerontologist, 24*, 144-148.

Sussman, M. B. (1976). The family of older people. In R. H. Binstock and E. Shanas (Eds.), *Handbook of aging and the social sciences* (pp. 218-243). New York: Van Nostrand Reinhold.

Thomas, P. D., Hunt, W. C., Garry, P. J., Hood, R. B., Goodwin, J. M., and Goodwin, J. S. (1983). Hearing acuity in a healty elderly population. *Journal of Gerontology, 38*, 321-325.

Troll, L. E. (1971). The family in later life: A decade review. *Journal of Marriage and the Family, 33*(4), 263-290.

Troll, L. E., Miller, S. J., and Atchley, R. C. (1979). *Families in later life.* Belmont, CA: Wadsworth.

Webster, J. C., Humes, H. W., and Lichtenstein, M. (1950). San Diego County Fair hearing survey. *Journal of Acoustical Society of America, 22*, 473-483.

White House Conference on Aging. (1981). *Report of the Technical Committee on Creating an Age-Integrated Society: Implications for the Family,* Washington, DC: Department of Health and Human Services.

Whitelaw, G. M., and Oyer, H. J. (1985). Effects of a concentrated program of education on the attitudes of hearing impaired adults. *Journal of Rehabilitation of the Deaf, 8*(1), 19-22.

Chapter 10
Developing SHHH, a Self-Help Organization

Howard E. Stone

I have been severely hearing impaired since I was 19, profoundly so since age 49. Mine is a noise-induced sensorineural loss with a hearing threshold of 110 dB in both ears. In 1975 I retired after a successful career of 25 years with the Central Intelligence Agency, including service in many countries in the Middle-East, Africa, and Asia and a period as chief of station in Italy.

For two years following my retirement, I helped to set up medical health centers for alcoholic priests and nuns. I then visited various organizations of and for deaf people, seeking to work in programs for the hard of hearing. There were none. I offered to develop some, but the organizations were not interested. They often referred to the millions of hearing-impaired people in justifying their programs, but their resources were directed at the smaller group of deaf people.

Some argued that partially deafened people have no real problem if they use a hearing aid. As a long-time hearing aid user, I knew that was not true. Of approximately 12 million people who could probably benefit from amplification, fewer than 2 million wore aids. But the comment I heard most frequently was, "You cannot organize hard-of-hearing people. They just will not respond."

At a meeting of the Alexander Graham Bell Association for the Deaf, I met William Paschell, who had an audio loop with which I heard better than I had in 34 years. Through him, I met an excellent local group of hard-of-hearing people, many of whom aspired to form a national organization, Consumers Organization for the Hearing Impaired (COHI).

Founded in 1977, COHI was having difficulties. I felt that hard-of-hearing people should not only join an organization but be involved in its activities. The purposes of COHI were too technical to permit that, and its name seemed more appropriate to the 1960s than the 1980s. No one worked full-time for it and no one put up the money necessary to form a genuine organization. All told, I concluded that the outlook of COHI was too limited.

John Gardner, founder of Common Cause, advised me to establish an independent organization devoted to self-help. I began recruiting friends and started an eight-week experiment in a local church, providing an audio loop and instructing people in its use.

In October, 1979, a story about my CIA experiences appeared on the front page of *The Wall Street Journal.* The formation of SHHH was mentioned only briefly; nonetheless, the hundred letters I received were all interested in SHHH. This response spurred me to proceed.

THE CONCEPT

SHHH was to be a membership organization of hearing-impaired people that would treat them as adults. Local chapters would have great autonomy. The national office would offer information about methods and tools of communication; members would decide for themselves how to use it. We would focus first on the human spirit and only later on hearing impairment, treating it as simply one more life crisis. The preamble to the SHHH Constitution reads:

> We are people who do not hear well, but are not deaf. We tend, increasingly, to be isolated. The existing pattern of community life lacks both means of communication and institutions for us to solve our special problems and live normal lives. For too long, too many of us have accepted a loneliness we are unable to explain to our friends or even to our families.
>
> We do not believe this situation is inevitable. We believe we can help one another, be helped, and live active, healthy lives. Because our hearing loss affects those close to us, we and they must do everything possible to improve communication. Our primary purpose, then, is to educate ourselves, our relatives and our friends about the cause, nature, complications and possible remedies of hearing loss.
>
> We believe that joy in sharing; strength in association; empathy and fellowship with peers; and a chance to help others who are in the same situation, is a way to begin.
>
> Therefore, in the conviction that by working together we can develop the realization that we are not alone, we have established "Self Help for Hard of Hearing People, Inc." to further our common welfare . . . .

ORGANIZATION

I chose a logo and had stationery and 10,000 copies of a brochure printed. A law firm volunteered to handle our incorporation free, and SHHH was incorporated in Maryland in November, 1979. My wife Alice

Marie, my son Michael, and I were the founders and officers, with other directors drawn from a broad group of interested persons. A second telephone line and a TTY were installed in the lower level of our home, which was rearranged as an office; a post office box and mailing permit were obtained, and an application was submitted for tax exemption. SHHH was open for business.

One evening, I received a telephone call. "Rocky, my name is Dick Schweiker and I like what you are doing. How can I help?" As senior Senator from Pennsylvania, Richard S. Schweiker was the ranking minority member of the Subcommittee on the Handicapped of the Committee on Labor and Human Resources. He agreed to arrange a hearing on the needs of hard-of-hearing as well as deaf people. I helped with the staff work and was the first witness at the February 6, 1980, hearing. *

TRAVEL

When a speaking engagement is made, I contact persons in several cities en route to arrange media coverage and meetings and to distribute brochures and membership forms. For example, a February, 1980, trip to Louisiana, Texas, and Georgia led to eight talks, several meetings with community leaders, 15 television and radio appearances, and good press coverage. I paid all the expenses.

In the last three years, I have spoken in 24 states and in Canada and Australia. Chapters have been formed in all but three of the places I visited and a national office has been established in Australia.

MEDIA AND MEMBERSHIP

Media attention is linked to membership. When SHHH was incorporated, I sent a short article to hundreds of news and magazine outlets around the country. We seek at least one major media event a month. Sometimes the media come to SHHH; sometimes, we go to them.

The June-July 1980 issues of *Modern Maturity* (circulation 8.5 million) contained a 125-word item reporting the birth and goals of SHHH and giving our address. We received 2,500 inquiries. Fortuitously, the first issue of our journal, *Shhh*, appeared in June; Walter T. Ridder of the Knight/

---

* See *Oversight on programs for the deaf and hearing impaired, 1980.* Hearing before the Subcommittee on the Handicapped of the Committee on Labor and Human Resources, U.S. Senate, 96th Cong., 2nd Session, February 6, 1980.

Ridder newspaper chain had financed 5,000 copies. Inquirers received a sample copy, brochure, and membership form. I wrote many personal replies in longhand. A group of friends and volunteers met regularly at our home to stuff, seal, and address envelopes and sort them by zip code to save postage. Our membership began to grow.

Membership cost $7 a year (raised to $10 in 1985). The Board of Directors questioned our ability to function with such a low fee. I argued that many elderly people are on fixed incomes and that hard-of-hearing people are not joiners. To succeed, we had to offer them high value.

Other magazines, such as *The Disabled American Veteran*, began to print my short article. When a magazine gives the dues and address of SHHH, many readers send checks, which reduces the cost of solicitation and provides immediate income.

William Neill, a Public Broadcasting System producer, wanted to produce three one-hour television programs on hearing loss; we worked together on them. Two have been completed. One was shown in 1982, the second in May 1984, and the third is scheduled for 1985. SHHH is listed in the credits.

By the summer of 1980, I was still the only full-time SHHH staff member. Volunteers worked 4 to 6 hours a week and groups were enlisted for major mailings. Ten or 12 volunteers would gather after working hours in the office of a law firm or insurance company and type addresses on master forms that were run through the firm's copy machine to produce labels. The reward was a wine and cheese party. As SHHH gained more public attention, my financial outlays rose.

1981 WHITE HOUSE CONFERENCE ON AGING

A White House Conference on Aging is held every ten years. In 1961, hearing-impaired people had been disregarded. In 1971, deaf but not hard-of-hearing people received some attention. The 1981 conference was being planned without consideration of either group. In October 1980, Arthur Fleming, who had chaired the 1971 conference, arranged a meeting for me with the conference staff. For two hours, I explained why the hearing loss of older Americans merited special attention. Jerome Waldie, the staff director, asked if I could organize a mini-conference on elderly hearing-impaired people and produce a report by February. I accepted.

Eight organizations agreed to sponsor the conference but only three contributed more than their name. The American Speech-Language-Hearing Association provided office space, a WATTS line, secretarial help, copy facilities, and a $1,500 loan for brochures and mailing. The National Association of the Deaf and the Alexander Graham Bell Association for the Deaf helped to defray expenses for interpreters. A friend and I called professionals around the country to seek their participation; without exception, they were most cooperative. We offered to pay the expenses of consumers invited to attend. The manufacturers of four major sound systems provided free equipment. At the conference, held January 11-13, 1981, in a Washington hotel, a group of loyal volunteers served as staff; I chaired the meeting and wrote the report. Although the National Institute on Aging provided a $5,000 research grant, we went deeply into debt until the Administration on Aging finally awarded SHHH $17,000 for the conference.

The conference report* stated that "hard of hearing people were much less informed than the deaf on subjects of vital importance to them." The conference recommended the following actions:

1. Publication of a consumers' guide to alternative hearing devices listing what is available, where to find it, what it costs, and how it is used.

2. Development and conduct of programs for service providers and consumers on hearing devices, alternative communication methods, and related information.

3. Assistance to local and state organizations (such as area agencies on aging, service clubs, and libraries) to provide audio-visual information and demonstration centers for the hearing impaired.

4. Encouragement of captioned public television programs.

SHHH mailed the mini-conference report, with a membership form on the back page, to 30,000 people. Although immediate response was small, the forms have been coming back for more than two and a half years. Most persons with an acquired hearing loss are slow to react to news that there is an organization to help them. Skepticism, resignation, denial, an attitude of "going it alone" is widespread. But slowly, more and more hearing-impaired people *are* responding to SHHH.

MEDIA SUCCESS AND FAILURE

In June, 1981, the television show "Over Easy" taped a segment on hearing impairment with Mary Martin and Jim Hartz as hosts and Florence Henderson, John Darby, and myself as guests. The show aired four times in two years. SHHH received 2,500 inquiries after each of the first two shows

---

* White House Conference on Aging (1981). *Report of the mini-conference on elderly hearing impaired people.* Washington, DC: U.S. Government Printing Office.

and 1,500 and 1,200, respectively, after the next two; 10 to 15 per cent of respondents became members.

By the end of 1981, SHHH had more than tripled its membership, but funds were low and we had trouble keeping abreast of the mail. With the help of the Advertising Council and Paul Higgins, who donated the services of his New York advertising firm Harrison and Higgins, I invested $18,000 in a three fifths of a page advertisement in *Modern Maturity*, the magazine of the American Association of Retired Persons. Estimating that over half of the magazine's 15 million readers had some hearing loss, I expected thousands of new SHHH members; only 300 materialized. SHHH is still in debt to Harrison and Higgins.

HELP ARRIVES

Early in 1982, Joan Kleinrock, who had been doing some work for SHHH at home, began coming to the office regularly. Now the mail could be serviced and the phone answered, referrals made and advice given while I was away. A 124-page Chapter Manual was completed and sent to organizers around the country.

The preceding October, Patricia Ann Clickener, an advertising executive with a profound hearing loss, had visited SHHH for a day. She organized chapters in the Chicago area and rented a TTY for frequent contact with the national office. She not only paid the costs of her work but generated $10,000 for SHHH through her donations and matching funds. (Walter Ridder and the Stone family were the only Founder members up to that time.)

In October 1982, after extensive preparations, I visited Australia, giving 34 talks and TV and media interviews in 17 days. An Australian National Office of SHHH resulted.

At the suggestion of a board member, manufacturers of amplification devices were asked to sponsor an issue of our journal for $2,500, which covered half the cost of printing and mailing 15,000 copies. In exchange, the firm received a full-page advertisement or statement on the back page.

THE FORWARD LEAP

In 1983, two more full-time volunteers joined the staff: Carol Lingley, who serves as office manager and receptionist, and Patricia Ann Clickener, who became SHHH vice-president.

As my home basement was becoming crowded and limiting, we took the risk of moving, in February 1983, to 2,000 square feet of modern office space at 4848 Battery Lane, Bethesda, Maryland 20814, just a block off the heavily traveled Wisconsin Avenue corridor near the National Institutes of Health. To economize, we built our own bookcases and storage cabinets, bought used furniture, and we received other items as gifts. As a result, the total cost of office appointments was under $1,500. Nonetheless, the rent, telephones, and equipment represented a substantial, continuing overhead cost.

CURRENT STATUS

Our increased staff enabled us to undertake more publications and services. Pat Clickener completed a Communications Access chart that compares the four major types of listening systems for large facilities such as churches, theaters, and auditoriums, enabling purchasers to choose the one best suited to their needs. With the help of Gwenyth Vaughan and Kirk Lightfoot, six pamphlets on assistive listening devices and systems were prepared. The foregoing publications are for sale; others were distributed free, such as a 40-page report on our first four years and a report on noise for a SHHH hearing conservation project aimed at schoolchildren in the first six grades. We also started work on an ombudsman program for hearing-impaired people in nursing homes.

A questionnaire on hearing loss, prepared by the Gallaudet Research Institute, was inserted in the January-February, 1984, issue of *Shhh*; over 1,600 responses, rich in information and suggestions, will help us to better understand and serve our members.

As of February, 1984, SHHH had 6,500 members: about 300 were libraries and organizations and the remainder were individuals; most were hearing impaired, but a number were relatives or friends of deafened persons, audiologists, teachers, or other professionals working with the hearing impaired. We hope that our membership will rise to over 11,000 by the end of 1984.

Our finances are weak because of the need for immediate outlays on new and expanded activities, but we should be out of debt by the end of 1984. If our efforts to obtain corporate and foundation support succeed, we hope to start paying our staff in 1985.

STRENGTHS AND PROBLEMS

The major strengths of SHHH are that it serves clearly defined needs. Our journal is popular and its positive philosophy gives courage and hope to many. Our local chapters bring people together to help each other, to share experiences and concerns, and to overcome the isolation so many deafened persons feel. The chapters and *Shhh News*, our chapter newsletter, also link members to the national office and help to implement SHHH programs in the local community. Our devoted full-time staff and part-time volunteers have been indispensable to the organization's success.

However, our reliance on volunteers is also a weakness. The full-time staff cannot be expected to contribute their work forever, and there are many activities necessary to the efficient, daily functioning of an office which part-time volunteers cannot be relied on to do. Volunteers must be enticed and persuaded; hired personnel may be instructed. SHHH lacks personnel with the time and experience to raise funds from foundations, members, and other sources. And the organization is in a genuine dilemma: to increase the membership, dues have been kept very low, but that does not yield the income needed to cover expenses and serve members adequately.

To encourage member participation, we suggest open chapter meetings and the creation of an atmosphere welcoming to all. But that can also create problems. For example, in one group deaf persons are in a majority; in another, a significant percentage; and many others have a few deaf members. They are often quick to speak up; unfortunately, because those who are deaf from birth or childhood may have speech difficulties, it can be difficult for lipreaders to understand them. Some sign as they talk, which can distract lipreaders to whom signing is new. Some view SHHH as a social outlet for the deaf. But SHHH was formed because hard-of-hearing people had no outlet of their own, no club or community center where they could come together to relax and communicate in comfort, not to engage in debates, conflict, and dissension. Deaf members are welcome so long as they accept SHHH's purposes and philosophy, remembering that SHHH was founded for hard-of-hearing people and seeks primarily to serve them.

The various types and degrees of hearing loss often pose communication problems. Most of our members are speech readers; few want or need to learn sign language, since their main need is to communicate with hearing people. Because of presbycusis or poor discrimination, all cannot benefit from assistive devices. The formation of small groups with similar hearing impairments, using whatever communication methods are best suited to their condition, may be the best solution.

Employed and retired persons have different needs and interests. The former want to keep their jobs and to satisfy their supervisors about their ability to do their work well. The problems of hearing television, concerts, movies, and phone conversations or communicating in a noisy setting are shared by all persons with a given type of hearing loss, regardless of age.

PROSPECTS

John Gardner has said that "SHHH has accomplished in four years what it takes most organizations ten years to accomplish." *

At present, aside from the small and technically-oriented Consumers Organization for the Hearing Impaired, there is no membership organization comparable to SHHH. However, SHHH may compete in certain activities with the celebrities employed by the Better Hearing Institute (BHI) sponsored by the hearing health industry. The National Association for Speech and Hearing Action (NASHA), an arm of the American Speech-Language-Hearing Association, calls itself a consumer organization and invites hearing-impaired persons to join. Both groups are useful; SHHH has good relations with both and can cooperate with them in many areas, while retaining the independence necessary to criticize them, when necessary.

Gallaudet College has shown a significant recent interest in deafened adults. A publication of the National Association of the Deaf has instituted a column on deafened adults. New groups are forming in California for adults who have lost or are losing their hearing. At SHHH's suggestion, a Congressman recently changed the title of legislation he has proposed from "National Deaf Awareness Week" to "National Hearing Impaired Awareness Week."† Awareness of and interest in acquired hearing loss is mounting, which augurs well for hearing-impaired people.

What should be the goals of SHHH as it grows in numbers, importance, and influence?

SHHH must maintain a personal touch regardless of its size. Individuals must remain our first priority.

SHHH should advocate legislation for deaf as well as hard-of-hearing people. United, the two groups can achieve more than will be possible if they are divided, and legislation that helps one group can also help the other.

SHHH should also work closely with industry to improve the quality and economy of remedial aids; help hearing people who are abused, victimized or defrauded; press for more research on the prevention and treatment of hearing loss; raise funds and award grants for research in neglected areas; sponsor forums and provide information on hearing health; endorse and help to implement policies to integrate hard-of-hear-

---

* Remarks to the SHHH staff, March, 1983.

† The bill was introduced by Congressman Frank J. Guarini (D—NJ) too late in the 1983 session to pass.

ing persons better into our society and work force; provide materials and services to help hard-of-hearing persons and their relatives and friends to accommodate better to each other; strive to enrich the lives of hard-of-hearing people with varied activities suited to their condition and preferences.

SHHH could not have been born, nurtured, and developed without the help of hundreds of people. Hearing people have helped greatly, but hearing-impaired people have carried the major load at both national and local levels.

The conclusion I draw from the experience of SHHH is: Do not rely on others or the government; act on your own and with your friends, and be prepared to pay the cost in money and time. Do not be afraid to gamble, for those who risk little, gain little.

PART IV
REVIEWING THE ISSUES

Chapter **11**

Psychosocial Aspects of Hearing Loss in Adulthood

Laurel E. Glass

A deaf colleague commented recently that it was difficult for him to remember that there are two major populations of older hearing-impaired persons: the deaf who are growing old and the old who are growing deaf. Although the biological effects of aging are similar, the emotional, social, and behavioral effects of hearing impairment in each population differ markedly. The old who are losing hearing are familiar to the "hearing world"—there are so many of them! However, their problems are essentially alien to persons deaf from infancy, who understand the difficulties of negotiating the hearing world but not the experience of losing hearing.

I am the hearing daughter of a mother who became severely hearing-impaired in midlife. She dealt with that impairment as realistically as possible, using amplification, lipreading, and other adaptations. Sign language was not one, because in her generation educators did not recognize it as a valid language. Due to her progressive hearing loss, she changed jobs in her mid-forties and retired early in her sixties when the hearing loss had become too handicapping. Before her death at 80, she could not hear even shouted speech. Thus, I lived for many years with someone undergoing the trauma of progressive impairment.

In reviewing some of the issues examined in preceding chapters, I will consider, successively, the impact of acquired hearing loss on the person who is losing hearing; the impact on family members and friends; interventions that may help those who are losing hearing and their families; and, lastly, some political issues.

PREVALENCE OF ADVENTITIOUS LOSS

The number of adults with an acquired hearing loss is very large. Even among the severely deaf, three fourths experienced their loss after the age of 17 (Schein and Delk, 1974). Although slightly less than 1 per cent of the population is profoundly deaf, the proportion with a significant hearing loss is much larger, especially among older adults. Noticeable hearing loss for high tones commonly occurs in persons only in their early thirties, at a younger age in men than in women (Corso, 1963). While the demographic data are neither abundant nor coherent (Chapter 1, pp. 5, 13; Ries, 1982), it is apparent that at least 1 in 4 persons over 64 has some trouble hearing. Some studies of the old-old in nursing home populations place the proportion as high as 9 in 10 (Chafee, 1967; Miller and Ort, 1965).

The Health Interview Survey (HIS) estimated that, in 1977, 7.2 million people had a bilateral hearing loss; the Health Examination Survey (HES), that 11.5 million had difficulty understanding speech. Unfortunately, the HIS and HES estimates cannot be compared directly. However, all population data indicate that the prevalence and severity of hearing impairment increases with age.

REACTIONS TO DEAFNESS

Adventitious hearing loss is not benign. Jack Ashley writes precisely; he does not use words carelessly (Chapter 4). Yet, note the phrases and words he uses about hearing loss: "thunderbolt," "shattering beyond belief," "devastating," "disastrous," "plummeting hopes," "tortured," "despair," "misery," "appalling change," "bleak," "desolating sense of loss," "I was painfully and permanently aware," "lifelong burden," "grievous hearing loss." These are not casual words from a casual man. Moreover, he writes them in the midst of a remarkable career in Parliament.

Conveyed by Ashley's paper, the writing of others who became deaf as adults (Elliott, 1978; Schatzki, 1978), the comments of professionals working with deafened adults (Levine, 1960; Luey, 1980; Ramsdell, 1978), and some of the research summarized by Meadow-Orlans (Chapter 3; see also Orlans and Meadow-Orlans, 1984, 1985) are the realities of loss, anger, grief, hopelessness, despair, deficit, and deprivation. Becoming deaf is experienced first as a *loss*. There is no respite; the newly deafened must continually cope; silence and adaptation never cease.

Contrast these feelings with those of prelingually deaf persons. At the 1983 meeting of the Medical Commission of the World Federation of the Deaf in Sicily, deaf participants repeatedly challenged the speakers, "Why do you speak of deafness as a disease?" Prelingual deaf persons evidently experience it as a *difference* rather than a deficit or disability—except when it interferes with work, promotion, or social activity.

Becker's (1980) study of 100 members of an aging prelingual deaf group emphasizes the bondedness of the intimate "deaf community." Many share a common experience in residential schools for the deaf and identify closely with the small prelingually deaf population. The vast majority employ the same sign language in old age as in their youth. Their fingers may grow arthritic and less precise, but their language and ability to communicate remain intact. The profound loss of contact that afflicts so many hearing people as they age does not trouble those who became deaf as children or never knew what hearing is.

For those with adult onset hearing loss, the age at which that loss begins and the rate at which it progresses are significant. A sudden loss due to disease, drugs, injury or other cause is traumatic. There is no time to acquire coping skills or get used to the idea of deafness. However, the condition persists and, as the difficult initial adjustments are made, the skills acquired remain useful.

In contrast, a gradual hearing loss is insidious and the condition is commonly denied for a surprisingly long time. It may first become evident in conversation with friends or family (see p. 123)—for example, "I told you that"; "I thought you understood"; "You don't pay attention"; or "You can hear when you want to." Finally, someone says, "You're getting deaf."

Family members, who are tired, hurried, and attending to other things, may be annoyed and impatient with someone who does not hear them. Even when the hearing impairment is acknowledged and the individual seeks help, the situation continues to deteriorate. Many persons experiencing a progressive hearing loss will say, "I could use the phone but could not hear from the other room, and then I found I could not use the phone." Or, "I used to hear my son but not my grandchildren, and now I can't hear my son." They accept a degree of loss and adjust to it. Then their hearing gets worse, and somehow they must cope again.

Most older persons who are losing hearing do so slowly. Repeatedly exposed to situations in which the information they receive is incomplete and confusing, they respond inappropriately. They must pay close attention to speakers. They must face the reality of a personal deficit and frequent failure of communication. No matter how hard they try, how tired or angry they feel, their hearing grows worse. Understandably, such cycles of loss, adjustment, and further loss are seriously stressful and often depressing. In one study of 7,000 persons representative of the population of Alameda County, California, depression and low quality of life were twice as common among hearing-impaired as hearing persons, and more common among hearing-impaired persons over age 54 than among those younger.

Hearing loss adds gravely to the other losses that older persons experience: the death of spouse, siblings, and friends; the loss of work, income, health, and mobility; the separation from familiar surroundings and perhaps from relatives and friends with a change of residence. Technological and social change may cause the loss of a world they knew. The loss of fittedness, freedom and community experienced by aging persons is aggravated for those who also lose their hearing. They lose the ability to acquire new information, to meet new people easily, to enter new situations comfortably and make their place in them. Perhaps the worst loss is the inability to share their thoughts and feelings readily and quietly. Who asks for your opinion or advice or shares theirs with you when you cannot hear what they say?

MUTABILITY OF AGE-ASSOCIATED LOSSES

A straight-line decline in physiological function with age occurs in several organ systems. However, not all age-related changes are inevitable and irreversible. Normal age-associated decline must be separated from the effects of illness and disease. Systems age at different rates, and their aging is assessed in different ways. A rapidly progressive change may kill before a slowly progressive, age-related change becomes a problem (Ludwig and Smoke, 1982). Yet nonlethal changes may interfere with the quality of life more than do the killing changes.

Since the straight-line graphs generally report cross-sectional data, cohort differences may be interpreted erroneously as age-related declines in function (Riley and Bond, 1983). Twenty year olds have more years of education than 65 year olds; obviously, that is due to historical or cohort factors, not age. Biological examples are more complex. A cohort of 20 year olds is taller than one of 70 year olds of the same race and social status. The difference represents both generational (cohort) and biological (intrinsic) factors. Young cohorts are taller than old ones were at the same age. In fact, 70 year olds are shorter than they themselves were 30 years before because of anatomical changes in the thickness of cartilaginous discs between their vertebrae. Thus, while age-associated changes may be intrinsic to the process of becoming old, they may also reflect generational—that is, mutable—differences in the aging person's cohort.

Sensorineural hearing loss in middle and later life probably represents such a mix of causal variables, some inherent in the physiology of auditory aging and some related to cohort, due to the accumulation of macro- and micro-assaults by noise, drugs, food contaminants, and other insults (Corso, 1977).

Anatomical changes have been described within the cochlea of older, hearing-impaired persons, especially in the stria vascularis and hair cells (Schuknecht, 1964; Johnsson and Hawkins, 1979). Decreased numbers of cells and fibers have been observed in the auditory nerve, brain stem tracts, and auditory cortex of elderly hearing-impaired individuals (Feldman and Vaughan, 1979). However, it is not understood why these lesions occur at different rates or why they occur where they do. Hearing loss in old age may not be "normal"; it may result in part from unnoticed, life-long insults, some of which may be preventable.

However, part of the complex etiology of hearing loss in old age may indeed reflect normal, or "natural," changes in the physiology of cochlear reception, neural transmission, and brain stem and cortical processing of auditory stimuli (Ordy, Brizzee, Beavers, and Medart, 1979). Older persons do not seem to process degraded, speeded, or slowed speech as well as younger persons, probably for physiological, not attitudinal, reasons (Bergman, 1980, 1983; Pickett, Bergman, and Levitt, 1979). Older people have more difficulty understanding reverberated speech. They have a higher incidence of tinnitus, which can be very troubling. Ironically, along with decreased sensitivity to sound, recruitment renders some tones painfully loud. Such symptoms are probably more associated with the biology of aging than with cohort changes.

The crucial points are that (1) some components of sensorineural hearing loss in old age may not be inevitable but may result from unknown and potentially controllable factors; (2) components intrinsic to the genetics and physiology of an aging organism and their effects can be ameliorated but not cured; and (3) astute research is needed to define which components are inevitable and which are not.

FAMILY RESPONSES

Schlesinger (Chapter 7) speaks of the implications of *power* and *powerlessness* for hearing-impaired or aging persons. Kyle, Jones, and Wood (Chapter 8) speak of *control* and suggest that "loss of control in the negotiated balance within the family" is a major problem for persons who are losing hearing. Implicit in the chapters by the Ashleys (Chapters 4 and 5) are issues of *independence* and *dependence*.

Such issues relate intimately to the individual's success or failure in adjusting to hearing loss and in responding to the efforts of family members and friends to help. To recognize the tensions—for example the need to retain independence and yet also to accept a degree of dependence—and to operate consciously within those paradoxical realities may be the difference between success and failure in coping with hearing loss. It is around these tensions that the problems of interacting with family and friends cluster. As previously noted, I am the daughter of a deafened mother. I also share a home with two adults, one of whom is deafened. Clearly, acquired deafness has a major effect on family function.

Pauline Ashley observed that her two older daughters were not as comfortable with their father's sudden hearing loss as the youngest, who was especially close to her father; she says little more about their reactions. Surely, their father's loss precipitated another traumatic loss for these children. Immediately after the blow fell, both parents struggled to grasp the problem and then to cope with it. Fortunately, Mrs. Ashley's mother and sister helped to care for the children. Nonetheless, during that period, the older girls effectively lost more of their father than did their sister, for she was so young she did not distinguish the father who had heard from the father who now did not hear.

Consider more common situations in which an adult loses hearing. How do family members react? Except for the report in this volume by Kyle and his colleagues (who focus on the hearing-impaired person) and the Oyers' thoughtful analysis (Chapter 9), researchers have paid little attention to the family constellation.

When talking to a lipreader, I speak more slowly and simply; I hesitate to express complex ideas and feelings. When I come home tired, I may want to slur words and speak carelessly. With a hearing-impaired listener, I must speak carefully or not about complex ideas. Like Mrs. Ashley, I am selective. In part, that is due to my fatigue at the end of the day and, in part, to consideration for the hearing-impaired friend whose day is often more tiring than mine. It takes more effort to receive information with four senses than with five; family members know that.

Family activities change. We go to the symphony less often and to the ballet more often. We play bridge more. We watch captioned foreign films and rarely see American and English films; as our deaf family member observes, "Too many are relentlessly verbal." Many adjustments are required, but they are worth it if the family is to remain united.

Despite our efforts, we often fail. Too often, I do not repeat important information or check that it is understood, and our hearing-impaired family member may feel confused or isolated. One evening, we were to pick up a friend, have dinner at a restaurant, and then go to the circus. Leaving home late, we picked up the friend and then drove rapidly away from the restaurant. After a time, the deaf family member said mildly, "I thought we had dinner reservations." "Yes, but first we have to mail something." We had verbally decided, in the dark, how to handle the problem of the letter and the restaurant but had neither signed nor written an explanation.

This kind of thing happens too often, although hearing loss is usually recognized and respected in our home. It probably occurs more often in families who are less aware of the implications of this disability. The hearing feel guilty and the hard-of-hearing feel left out. This dyad may be inevitable, even in good and accepting relationships between the deaf and the hearing.

Table 8-3 (p. 129) shows that hard-of-hearing persons feel that their family does not really understand their difficulties. A deaf friend and I read the manuscript of that chapter. I read it first and wrote in the margin that I thought the authors should also have interviewed the family members, who were probably more aware of these difficulties than the hearing-impaired person realized. My deaf friend looked at that and did not comment; she did not agree.

There is a great need for research on the varied changes in family relations that occur as one member loses hearing. Successful coping probably requires unsuspected adaptations which are costly to all family members.

When an adult is losing hearing, changes occur in the way the family functions, although they may not seem important if they sustain a valued relationship. This is one of the strongest messages conveyed by Pauline Ashley. Whatever her husband needed from her—human support, help with lipreading, interpreting, phone answering—she was prepared to give. She did not feel "put upon"; her relationship with her husband was worth it.

In many families, this is unequivocally the case; the relationship is, indeed, worth it. Nonetheless, after a spouse loses hearing, many marriages end in divorce (Hunter, 1978).

COMMUNICATION AFTER HEARING LOSS

The chapters in this volume implicitly, if not explicitly, recognize that any form of communication is appropriate and good if it helps hearing-impaired persons to share information and feelings with others. The key idea is communication.

Many older persons reject hearing aids and other recommended rehabilitation measures (Chapter 6). Hearing aids irritate as well as help, although currently available aids may irritate less than those of the past. As a population, we may now have a higher tolerance for noise than in earlier days: it is so omnipresent. If this is true, newly aging cohorts may use hearing aids more readily, because they can better tolerate the irritation of the magnified noise.

Many studies indicate that older people tend to deny hearing loss and may not use a hearing aid after buying it (Alpiner, 1982). A recent dissertation by Nguyen (1984) confirmed this. More unexpected, however, were Nguyen's data suggesting that older persons may not receive hearing health care because the examiner fails to recommend follow-up by a physician. Also unexpected was her finding that denial or acceptance of hearing loss had no significant correlation with whether the patient accepted rehabilitation and hearing aid recommendations.

Nguyen is conducting further research into these findings. They remind us that stereotypic expectations of the behavior of older persons based on studies of aged cohorts from previous decades may inappropriately restrict research and treatment. Riley and Bond (1983) emphasized a point made in the preceding section of this chapter: aging, or at least how one ages, is mutable, and many changes attributed solely to aging also reflect personal and social responses to that biological phenomenon (see also Chapter 2). This is important to those who work or live with aging adults whose hearing is deteriorating.

Communication modes must be personally and socially *accessible*. To sign, wear a hearing aid, or use cued speech is to call attention to oneself and to a disability that is, or is felt to be, stigmatized (Herbst, 1983). It is easier to withdraw than to expose one's disability to the misunderstanding and insensitivity of others. Those with impaired hearing must be helped to supplement their communication skills as best they can so that they can remain active participants in our common world.

As noted, powerlessness and a feeling of loss of control are often aspects both of an "aging" and a "hearing loss" syndrome. Therefore, an important part of accessibility for older persons with an acquired hearing loss is the need to be affirmed and supported in their use of whatever communication devices and techniques they choose. If a hard-of-hearing person wants to lipread rather than to sign, or vice versa, that is her or his choice, not ours. We should advise the hearing impaired that if your families will write, write; if they will sign, sign; if they will learn cued speech, learn it; if they will do none of those, lipread and insist that they repeat until you understand. Communicate however and as best you can, but communicate.

Since at least 50 per cent of older adults will become hearing impaired, all middle-aged and old persons should be encouraged to practice lipreading while they have hearing, at least by watching the speaker's mouth. Remember—unlike a hearing aid, lipreading poses no problem with respect to appearance or stigma.

Any sign language can greatly enhance communication. However, to an adult who is losing hearing, American Sign Language (ASL) is more foreign than French or German. Not only are the syntax, grammar, body language, facial expressions, and hand positions difficult to learn, but hearing friends and family do not usually know or use it. When adults whose native language is English lose hearing, they remain culturally English-speaking and do not suddenly become part of the deaf community whose members have used ASL since childhood. To advise the person who was deafened as an adult to learn the new, complex grammar and syntax of ASL is to invite failure. However, it may be useful and practical for them and close family members to learn *some* Signed English and to spell out letters with their fingers.

A friend had a severe hearing loss diagnosed in her early twenties; since then, she has become profoundly deaf with virtually no testable auditory reception within the speech ranges. As her residual hearing failed, her lipreading grew worse and sign language became mandatory if she wished to communicate comfortably. However, ASL was a foreign language to her and she had difficulty learning it. As her hearing failed, she had supplemented her limited hearing with lipreading. Now, when profoundly deaf, she reads sign language much more fluently if she can supplement it with lipreading. If people use Signed English or Pidgeon Signed English, mouthing the words, she understands them well. Without lipreading, she understands Signed English less well. She uses ASL adequately, but is not fluent.

The disability of this well-trained, very intelligent, highly motivated, warmly relating woman becomes a handicap only when she must use her foreign second language, ASL. Her lipreading skill is then useless and her comprehension of sign language is less complete.

For most aging adults who are losing hearing slowly, Signed English may be accessible, although ASL is not. Unfortunately, in the San Francisco Bay Area and many other areas, ASL is at present the only manual language readily available. Few Signed English classes are offered.

The extensive linguistic research on ASL during the last two or three decades has advanced our understanding of its beauty, complexity, and integrity. Since the sign language and lipreading needs of persons losing hearing in adulthood are quite different from those of persons deaf from infancy (it is easier to pattern sign based on a language the person knows), research on adventitious deafness needs to focus on different questions, such as the following: How many words can be missed without losing meaning? How much information is lost by the hearing-impaired individual because speakers simplify language structure?

Research is also needed on many other aspects of hearing loss, such as the strains which it places on marriage and the family and why and how some deafened persons and their families do and do not cope.

HEARING LOSS AND POLITICS

The "deaf community" commonly refers to those deafened at birth or in childhood who share a common language (ASL), an education in residential schools for the deaf, and characteristic patterns of socialization and interaction which may be termed "the culture of the deaf." In contrast, persons who lose their hearing in adulthood are culturally hearing persons with a voiced and not a manual language. Each population has different characteristics and needs. Nonetheless, both share certain common needs—for example, for amplification; ways to use residual hearing; sign language or oral interpreters; captioning; and many other services which help them to work and live as minority members in a majority world.

Some needs conflict. Population statistics cited in support of the free TDD legislation in California included figures for the prelingually deaf, for adventitiously deafened adults, and for unilaterally or bilaterally hard-of-hearing persons. No wonder the demand for free TDDs was far less than projected; deafened adults did not know they might be eligible.

This example, and others not cited, suggests that the needs of aging, hearing-impaired persons must be addressed politically in an informed way. Cooperation with the prelingual deaf community is desirable when the needs of the two groups coincide. Negotiation, accommodation, and compromise are necessary when their needs diverge.

A pragmatic approach to such issues has been taken by SHHH (Self Help for Hard of Hearing People, Inc.) (Chapter 10) and some regional hearing societies. Recently, the American Association for Retired Persons has begun to address the problems of hearing loss in old age. Unless adventitiously deafened and hard-of-hearing persons are active in the political process, too little money will be designated for services for and research on their needs. Professional persons concerned with adventitious hearing loss should become politically literate and seek to make legislation and rehabilitative services informed and effective. Hearing loss in middle and later life will not cease to exist. It can become less handicapping if relieved by appropriate knowledge and services.

REFERENCES

Alpiner, J. G. (1982). Rehabilitation of the geriatric client. In J. G. Alpiner (Ed.), *Handbook of adult rehabilitative audiology* (2nd ed., pp. 160-208). Baltimore: Williams & Wilkins.

Becker, G. (1980). *Growing old in silence.* Berkeley: University of California Press.

Bergman, M. (1980). *Aging and the perception of speech.* Baltimore: University Park Press.

Bergman, M. (1983). Central disorders of hearing in the elderly. In R. Hinchcliffe (Ed.), *Hearing and balance in the elderly* (pp. 145-158). Edinburgh: Churchill Livingstone.

Berkman, L. F., and Breslow, L. (1983). *Health and ways of living: The Alameda County study.* New York: Oxford University Press.

Chafee, C. E. (1967). Rehabilitation needs of nursing home patients: A report of a survey. *Rehabilitation Literature, 28,* 377-381.

Corso, J. F. (1963). Aging and auditory thresholds in men and women. *Archives of Environmental Health, 6,* 56-62.

Corso, J. F. (1977). Auditory perception and communication. In J. E. Birren and K. W. Schaie (Eds.), *Handbook of the psychology of aging* (pp. 535-553). New

York: Van Nostrand Reinhold.

Elliott, H. H. (1978). Shifting gears. Paper presented at Workshop for Deafened Adults of the Hearing Society for the Bay Area and the Deaf Counseling, Advocacy and Referral Agency, San Francisco.

Feldman, M. L., and Vaughan, D. W. (1979). Changes in the auditory pathway with age. In S. S. Han and D. H. Coons (Eds.), *Special senses in aging: A current biological assessment* (pp. 143-162). Ann Arbor: University of Michigan, Institute of Gerontology.

Herbst, K. G. (1983) Psycho-social consequences of disorders of hearing in the elderly. In R. Hinchcliffe (Ed.), *Hearing and balance in the elderly* (pp. 174-200). Edinburgh: Churchill Livingstone.

Hunter, C. C. (1978). A pilot study of late deafened adults. Unpublished master's thesis, California State University, Northridge.

Johnsson, L. G., and Hawkins, J. R., Jr. (1979). Age-related degeneration of the inner ear. In S. S. Han and D. H. Coons (Eds.), *Special senses in aging: A current biological assessment* (pp. 119-135). Ann Arbor: University of Michigan, Institute of Gerontology.

Levine, E. (1960). Progressive and sudden hearing loss. In E. Levine (Ed.), *Psychology of deafness* (pp. 56-74). New York: Columbia University Press.

Ludwig, F. C., and Smoke, M. E. (1982). The measurement of biological age. *Gerontology, 1*, 27-37.

Luey, H. S. (1980). Between worlds: The problems of deafened adults. *Social work in health care, 5*, 253-265.

Miller, M., and Ort, B. (1965). Hearing problems in a home for the aged. *Acta Otolaryngologica, 59*, 33-44.

Nguyen, M. (1984). *Denial and follow-up as predictors of outcome among elderly clients screened in a hearing outreach program.* Unpublished doctoral dissertation, California School of Professional Psychology, Berkeley.

Ordy, J. M., Brizzee, K. R., Beavers, T., and Medart, P. (1979). Age differences in the functional and structural organization of the auditory system in man. In J. M. Ordy and K. R. Brizzee (Eds.), *Sensory systems and communication in the elderly* (pp. 153-166). New York: Raven Press.

Orlans, H., and Meadow-Orlans, K. (1984, September/October). Who are the members of SHHH? A report on the *Shhh* questionnaire. *Shhh, 5*, 3-5.

Orlans, H., and Meadow-Orlans, K. (1985, January/February). Responses to hearing loss: Effects on social life, leisure and work. *Shhh, 6*, 4-7.

Pickett, S. N., Bergman, M., and Levitt, H. (1979). Aging and speech understanding. In M. M. Ordy and K. R. Brizzee (Eds.), *Sensory systems and communication in the elderly* (pp. 167-186). New York: Raven Press.

Ramsdell, D. A. (1978). The psychology of the hard-of-hearing and the deafened adult. In H. Davis and S. R. Silverman (Eds.), *Hearing and deafness* (4th ed., pp. 499-510). New York: Holt, Rinehart and Winston.

Ries, P. W. (1982). *Hearing ability of persons by sociodemographic and health characteristics: United States.* National Center for Health Statistics. (Series 10, No. 140). Washington, DC: United States Government Printing Office.

Riley, M. W., and Bond, K. (1983). Beyond ageism: Postponing the onset of disability. In M. W. Riley, B. B. Hess, and K. Bond (Eds.), *Aging in society* (pp. 243-253). Hillsdale, NJ: Lawrence Erlbaum Associates.

Schatzki, L. M. (1978). If I knew then what I know now . . . . Paper presented at Workshop for Deafened Adults of the Hearing Society for the Bay Area and the Deaf Counseling, Advocacy and Referral Agency, San Francisco.

Schein, J. D., and Delk, M. T., Jr. (1974). *The deaf population of the United States.* Silver Spring, MD: National Association of the Deaf.

Schuknecht, H. F. (1964). Further observations on the pathology of presbycusis. *Archives of Otolaryngology, 80,* 369-382.

Chapter 12
Reflections on Adult Hearing Loss

Harold Orlans

Do numbers count? A very large number of persons suffer a significant hearing loss in mid-career or later life—one estimate gives a figure of 4.9 million in 1971 in the United States; estimates of the total number of Americans with some hearing loss range from 18.7 million to over 29.1 million. That is, 76 per cent of the estimated 6.4 million persons with serious bilateral hearing loss ("at best can hear shouted speech") lost their hearing after the age of 20 (see Table 1-9, p. 17). Ries (Table 1-1, p. 5) gives an estimate of 18.7 million in 1981. A careful restudy of Health and Nutrition Examination Survey data for 1971-75 yields estimates ranging from 7.7 to 43.5 million adults aged 25-74, depending upon the Hertz frequencies and decibel levels chosen to define "hearing impairment." Employing 1981 Occupational Safety and Health Administration criteria for hearing loss, the authors estimated its prevalence in 1971-75 as 8.4 to 27.8 per cent or 8.7 to 29.1 million persons aged 25 to 74 (Singer, 1982, p. 53).

Why has this vast population been scarcely noted by psychologists and social scientists, who study so many other groups? Why are there so few organizations that represent and serve their interests? Why do we know so little about feelings and conduct of these people; their personal, social, and occupational problems; and the different ways, good, poor, and tragic, by which they and their families adjust to their condition?

The hearing-impaired population is too heterogeneous to be studied easily and adequately. It includes the totally deaf and those with so slight a hearing loss they do not recognize it; those deafened in infancy and those deafened in old age; those whom a hearing aid can help and those who cannot be helped. It is no accident that the two best known segments of the hearing-impaired population, the prelingually deaf and the elderly deafened, are two of the most homogeneous.

Except for prelingually deaf persons, whose identity and condition are inseparable, many—perhaps most—hearing-impaired persons shrink from identifying with other deafened people. For long years they were part of the hearing world and they want to remain part of it, as best they can. They would rather be isolated in it than united in a deafened world. If people with poor eyesight or warts do not identify with one another, why should those with poor hearing? The leaders of Self Help for Hard of Hearing People are unusual persons who will not yield to affliction and have confronted, not evaded, their condition; those who join seek the relaxation and comfort of company "with whom you don't have to say you're sorry" (as Howard Stone put it at the 1983-84 Gallaudet seminar). *

Stone has suggested that a clinical approach, the search for extreme conditions to facilitate diagnosis, has led researchers to concentrate on the totally deaf and on deaf children who have severe needs, rather than the larger but more variegated hearing-impaired population. Surely, practical factors governing the economics and politics of research also operate. The greater homogeneity of the prelingually deaf and the concentration of children in schools for the deaf make them more accessible for study, although communication difficulties render them less so; their teachers, counselors, and parents want the information that scholars and publishers provide; and research grants and university appointments sustain the scholars. In time, as the main subgroups of the larger hearing-impaired population are better defined and understood, they will become more accessible to study through hearing-aid dealers, audiologists, lipreading classes, self-help groups, retirement centers, and nursing homes; a market will develop for information about them; and universities, professional associations, foundations, and research programs will help to generate that information.

THE DEGREE, RAPIDITY, AND AGE AT ONSET OF HEARING LOSS

If the degree of loss is the permeable or dense barrier between the individual and hearing society, the inescapable condition to which he or she must respond, character is a primary factor governing response. The responses of different individuals to comparable degrees of hearing loss can differ strikingly. Some grow irritable or morose; marriages can become strained or break. Some persons, with solid marriages, rely heavily upon their spouse's ears. Many withdraw to their homes and then withdraw again, within their families, or live alone and companionless. Some continue to function remarkably well; their lipreading skills, intelligence, even temper, directness, and, above all, will power compensate for their deafness. The sensitive or vain, who see themselves only in the mirror of society,

---

* Other unidentified quotations in this chapter are also drawn from participants' comments at the seminar.

suffer painfully from a loss which the confident, strong-willed, or thick-skinned disregard.

Persons with normal hearing are immersed in abundant sounds; some are distracting or aggravating—noises, sirens, loud music, a clock ticking, the tiny plop of a faucet, or the creaking of wood in a quiet room. If background noise presents a more acute problem to those with poor hearing, competing with the speech they seek to discern, the value of the sounds they still hear is heightened. Some who cannot understand speech with a powerful hearing aid may yet wear it throughout the day for the clues it gives to what is going on. Jack and Pauline Ashley stress how important was the "wisp of hearing" or the "scratch of sound" to his learning to lipread (see pp. 61 and 73). When that wisp went, "I appreciated the difference between the very hard of hearing and the totally deaf."

The nature and degree of residual hearing remain significant throughout the spectrum of hearing loss. Exasperating problems can arise with a relatively moderate but slowly growing loss that makes it possible to continue work as a teacher, nurse, secretary, salesman, or cabdriver, but an increasing strain and, in certain situations, danger.

Current survey instruments do not satisfactorily measure the nature of an individual's hearing loss and how well he or she functions with it. A good audiologist or otolaryngologist working with a social worker or psychologist can assess this quite well after detailed and repeated clinical examinations and inquiries. But the truncated hearing tests and questions employed in examination and interview surveys of large populations miss major pieces of the complex picture of hearing loss and adjustment to it. Thus, the Gallaudet Hearing Scale (see Figure 1-1) attempts to approximate measured decibel loss with answers to a series of questions about ability to understand or hear progressively louder sounds. Lacking anything better, the scale remains useful but inadequate, for hearing loss is not necessarily linear; many persons can hear soft speech better than loud. In addition, a good lipreader with a severe hearing loss can function better than a poor lipreader with a moderate loss.

Because the prevalence of hearing impairment rises rapidly with age, we are apt to think that most hearing-impaired persons are elderly. This is not the case. On one estimate, three fifths of persons with hearing loss were under 65. However, two thirds of the severely deafened were 65 or over (Table 12-1).

Information on age at onset is scanty but, plainly, many elderly persons with a serious hearing loss began to lose their hearing in childhood or as young adults. According to an analysis of the responses of 1,445 elderly persons with a serious loss to a questionnaire in the January-February 1984 issue of *Shhh*, 18 per cent had lost some hearing before they were 10; 28 per cent, before they were 20; and 40 per cent, before they were age 30.

Table 12-1. Number and Per Cent of Persons with Some and with Severe Hearing Loss, by Age, 1977

Hearing loss	Age			
	Total	3-44	45-64	65+
Number (thousands)				
All levels	12,849	3,558	4,238	5,053
At best can hear words shouted in ear	756	112	140	504
Per Cent				
All levels	100	28	33	39
At best can hear words shouted in ear	100	15	19	67

From Ries, P.W. (1982). *Hearing ability of persons by sociodemographic and health characteristics: United States* (Series 10, No. 140). National Center for Health Statistics. Washington, DC: U.S. Government Printing Office.

Hence, many must adjust and readjust to a condition that deteriorates slowly and irregularly over years or decades, not knowing how long their hearing will remain or how quickly it will fade.

Jack Ashley, whose hearing loss was sudden, called "creeping deafness . . . a very slow form of paralysis." Howard Stone found it frustrating and tormenting. In contrast, sudden loss is traumatic, "one of the most terrifying experiences" (Lehmann, 1954, p. 1481), like an amputation, a bomb blast, or a death. Norman Bethune, a 49 year old surgeon, suddenly became completely deaf, evidently from an angiospasm, during an operation behind the battlefield.

> He put down his scalpel, took off his gown, and left the operation room, ordering his assistant to finish the operation . . . . "He was deeply scared. He was listening for the singing of the birds, the sound of the wind. But in his ears there was only a satanic pounding, as if the blood was coursing through his head with the roar of a distant river. He asked himself: Would he never hear more music, no more voices of friends, no more sounds of fields, bugle calls, laughter? . . . . He saw himself in the operating room like a bird in a cage." (Allan and Gordon, 1952, p. 293)

However, because it is decisive, not lingering and ambiguous, denial is less lasting; the crisis must be confronted; shock, grief, and depression must be followed by accommodation.

The age at onset and, of course, the severity of the loss determine the likelihood of continued active participation in, or withdrawal from, hearing society. A mild loss may be functionally defined as one with which normal participation can continue (if necessary, with the use of a hearing aid) and a moderate loss, one with which hearing society remains paramount but greater breaks in communication arise. With a severe loss, the breaks become pronounced and with profound deafness, overriding.

When deafness is total and early, the child or adolescent usually will learn to sign and be educated in schools for deaf students. When deafness comes late, after retirement, an elderly person may maintain only such contact with society as his or her eyes and tongue permit. Those moderately deafened in their middle years face cruel and difficult choices and may struggle for years with themselves, their families, and their friends and colleagues before reaching a resolution of their practical and emotional problems, either by choice or, perhaps as often, by events.

THE CHOICES OF DEAFENED ADULTS

> ... deafness ... does not set a sharply defined line of demarcation between the things that the handicapped person should expect to be able to do and the things that are clearly beyond his reach. To establish this line for himself so as to avoid a retreat from what is still possible, and at the same time to avoid a useless struggle and defeat in trying to do the impossible: this is perhaps the most important problem in the adjustment of the deaf man. (Heider and Heider, 1941, p. 131)

The problem outlined in this quotation is primarily one of communication and sociability, of knowing what is said and of being able to respond at work or home, with friends or strangers. It is most difficult for those who must work with people (not machines or paper) they do not know under conditions they cannot control. Printers or computer programmers (traditional and modern occupations for deaf people), postal clerks manning mail-sorting machines, typists transcribing written copy, farmers, coal miners, bookkeepers, writers, craftsmen, painters, mechanics, carpenters, and gardeners need not change their jobs if they become hard of hearing. Doctors, chemists, or astronomers may continue working in a quiet office, laboratory, or observatory. But not salesmen, secretaries, stockbrokers, or reporters, who must use the phone; waitresses, teachers, social workers, or policemen, who must hear clearly in noisy settings; actors, supervisors, or interpreters, who must catch and respond immediately to the tone as well as the content of what is said.

People in jobs not requiring good hearing may remain in them, as their hearing fades, if they are effective and if their colleagues help out by repeating or writing instructions and taking or making phone calls. Others will have to change or modify their work—for example, a secretary may become a typist; a teacher, a tutor; a reporter, a writer; a lawyer, a legal researcher. Unhappily, the new work usually requires less skill or versatility, pays less, and has fewer prospects for advancement. Nonetheless, those without independent means or other forms of support must try to hang on, one way or another, until retirement. In one group of 682 elderly persons with severe hearing loss surveyed in 1984, the median age of retirement was 62.6, or the middle of the first year after which Social Security benefits could be drawn (Orlans and Meadow-Orlans, 1984, p. 4).

Even a modest hearing loss, especially the common sensorineural kind that does not just diminish but warps sound, gravely hampers relaxed and easy sociability, which depends on not just the meaning but also the context and inflection of words, quick repartee, interruptions, jokes, nuances, and word play. The hearing impaired person who can manage well with an old friend in a quiet room is utterly adrift in a convivial group where words and banter, shouts and laughter, wisecracks, puns, and guffaws resound. One line of careful speech the hearing-impaired person might follow; amid many voices flying about he or she is lost. What is fun for the hearing is torture for the deafened—snatches of words tossing in a hubbub of noise.

The slow, simplified, and careful conversation that poor hearing demands may contribute to the common complaint that deafness is equated with dumbness. Of course it is not; but deafness is, unfortunately, equated with stilted and impoverished conversation drained of many qualities that enrich and enliven normal speech. Except for those who sign or whose hearing is fully corrected by an aid, conversation between a deafened and a hearing person is seldom both full and relaxed; there are only varying degrees of patience, effort, and care; truncation and fatigue; tension and frustration; or silence.

Women apparently adjust to hearing loss better than men. Their loss tends to be somewhat less severe and occurs later (see p. 18); they tend to have less demanding jobs, which may be more readily replaced by more manageable ones; they may accept, or have accepted, a greater degree of dependency than men; and deafness requires fewer changes for housewives than for those who work outside the home. Some 52 per cent of the members of Self Help for Hard of Hearing People are women (not a high proportion for a group with an average age of 62), and they have been the most successful leaders of local chapters. Women, Howard Stone suggested, were not afraid of trying, whereas men, more accustomed to a position of control, are less likely to risk being hurt or embarrassed. And women, Jean Mulrooney said, were more prepared to admit their handicap. (If this is true, they should also be more inclined to wear a hearing aid.)

The strain of hearing, the danger of mishearing, the mischief, misfortune, or grief of not hearing, the aggravation of meeting people who assume you can hear must be endured at work. These pains and indignities need not be endured to the same degree during leisure hours, if they are spent at home or in activities that involve the hands, eyes, or legs rather than ears. There are countless activities available to a hearing-impaired person: he or she may knit, crochet, or weave; paint, sketch, sculpt, or photograph; write letters and read; play chess, cards, scrabble, or video games; garden or do household repairs; look after pets and plants; walk, bowl, or exercise; go to museums, exhibits, sporting events, the ballet, or foreign films with subtitles. Some, however, will avoid parties, noisy restaurants or bars; lectures, meetings, concerts, the theater, opera, movies; the radio or phonograph; the phone; and socializing, except in quiet with a good friend or relative.

Since the ability to socialize, to converse easily and casually in varied settings, is so threatened by a hearing loss, such a loss should be a greater affliction to a sociable, outgoing person than to a shy, introverted one who dislikes parties and prefers a quiet time at home. The strong, self-confident person who acts with assurance should manage hearing loss better than the sensitive person who will suffer mightily rather than speak up to announce his condition or change a seating arrangement. Assertiveness training has been suggested as a useful part of a rehabilitation program for the hearing-impaired (see DiMichael, 1983).

As hearing deteriorates, events render an accustomed style of accommodation unsatisfactory and a new style must be found. The events may be an inability to grasp a stranger's remarks, errors in understanding familiar speech, being quickly abandoned and isolated at gatherings, being reprimanded at work, losing a job, or finding a hearing aid less useful. The new accommodation may involve wearing an aid or getting a stronger one, taking a job where hearing is less important, retiring, or learning to lipread, to fingerspell, or to sign. Yet it is extraordinary how differently people can respond to the same condition and events. Some can go for years without acknowledging that they are hard of hearing and nonetheless adapt remarkably well to their loss. Indeed, Holly Elliott has argued that denial can be a positive help in coping.

> When I was 19 and a music major in college, an otologist told me that I was severely deaf, it would probably get worse, a hearing aid would not help, and I would have to learn to live with it. I felt anger—"Nobody's going to tell me what I can or can't do!"—and continued living as if I could hear . . . . I probably would not have had the strength to act as normally as I did if I had admitted and *felt* "I am deaf."
>
> For example, I continued directing choirs even after I lost the upper half of the piano keyboard. I heard the basses and patterned the rest in my mind. I lipread the sopranos and knew if they were off pitch by the expression on the tenors' faces—I always had very expressive tenors. If that was a "denial," it was also a positive way of coping that helped me to conduct sign language choirs after I lost the other half of the piano keyboard.

Most professionals dealing with hearing loss make the opposite argument, that an individual must acknowledge his or her condition before he or she can adjust satisfactorily to it. Surely, there are two kinds of adjustment processes: one occurs naturally, without conscious awareness and intellectualizing; the other requires conscious recognition and deliberate change. The conscious process is not necessarily superior, although it is necessary for certain purposes, such as getting a hearing test and a hearing aid. But awareness that one is becoming a kind of person one does not want to be can present an insurmountable obstacle to change. A realistic recognition of one's condition facilitates a good adjustment only if that recognition is accompanied by self-respect, not bitterness and self-hatred. *

Many people would rather not hear than identify with the hard of hearing by wearing an aid; would rather not hear with an aid than identify with the totally deaf by learning to lipread; and would rather lipread poorly than identify with prelingually deaf people by learning to sign. The idea of "stigma," the aversion to and casting off of disfigured members by society, has been widely invoked to explain this strange, strong resistance to appropriate and sensible adjustments. Goffman, who has discussed stigma perceptively, writes:

> The central feature of the stigmatized individual's situation . . . . is a question of . . . "acceptance." Those who have dealings with him fail to accord him the respect and regard which the uncontaminated aspects of his social identity have led them to anticipate extending, and have led him to anticipate receiving; he echoes this denial by finding that some of his own attributes warrant it. (1963, pp. 8-9)

As Goffman recognizes, a stigma is a condition invoking both social opprobrium and self-opprobrium, not just derogation by "normal" people but self-derogation by the stigmatized. The latter half of this equation is often disregarded, as it was in the Gallaudet seminar discussions. It is easier, in the company of deafened persons, to indict the callousness, cruelty, fear, stupidity, and indifference of innumerable ignorant members of "society" than to observe that society does not account for all the difficulties of hearing-impaired persons; that some of their greatest difficulties arise within themselves; and that, given the best conceivable conduct and attitudes by people who do and do not hear well, practical difficulties in communication, and their attendant social consequences, will remain.

The question of stigma, the balance between social and self distaste for deafness, arises in connection with the use of hearing aids. As is well known, a great many people who could benefit from an aid refuse to wear

---

* Holly Elliott, a clinical social worker who has counseled many deaf persons, spoke of a young prelingually deaf woman who visited her, "looked very intently at me and signed 'Teach me to love myself; I don't love myself now.' Rocky [Howard Stone] and SHHH are teaching hard-of-hearing people to love themselves. That is vital for all people to live contentedly, . . . but it is particularly difficult for those who do not [hear]."

one, and most of those who do choose an inconspicuous type worn behind or in the ear, rather than a more visible body type, which is sturdier, more powerful, and easier to use. One explanation is that they do not want to announce their disability and be stigmatized. Without an aid, they can pass for normal even though suffering, in consequence, the anxiety of pretending to hear and the small and large embarrassments, errors, and calamities that follow when their deception fails. In time, they may be the only one in their circle who does not see the failure. And when they too admit it, they may still refuse to wear an aid, preferring the status of a hard-of-hearing person who is otherwise "normal" or unmarred to one who posts a public notice of disfigurement.

An aid does not just help to correct a hearing loss; it notifies strangers and reminds the wearer of the loss. Since the inconspicuous aids that are so popular are deficient in both respects, it appears that the outlook of those who wear them remains in some ways comparable to that of the hearing-impaired people who do not. They regard a hearing aid as an unpleasant prosthesis, like a metal and plastic foot, and wear it naturally only after much use.

A simple explanation of the refusal to wear an aid may be offered that has nothing to do with stigma. We all cling to an image of ourselves that has little connection with the image others see. It is a perseveration, the residue in memory, habit, feeling, and character of days long past. Who, looking in the mirror, does not see, beneath the wrinkles, the lineaments of the same smooth features he or she has seen since youth—and what stranger sees anything but the wrinkles? We will not happily wear anything—a hat, dress, coat, ring, or tie—that does not fit the image we have of ourselves, which often has an element of self-flattery and illusion, that we are younger, thinner, or more attractive than is, in fact, the case. Why, then, having heard normally for so many years, should we suddenly attach a strange object to our ear?

No one, seeing Bernard Baruch—baronial, avuncular, and spotlessly groomed—holding forth to the press on a park bench or to Congressmen in a Congressional hearing room, with a large hearing aid held prominently in his hand or propped on the table before him, could imagine him suffering from a stigma. No one seeing Franklin Roosevelt or Ronald Reagan in command, genial and relaxed, could imagine either of them being stigmatized as crippled or hard of hearing. No one, seeing Jack Ashley or Howard Stone, the one outgoing and irrepressibly good-humored, the other even-tempered and businesslike, both self-assured and yielding nothing to their disability, can see them suffering from a stigma. Are these unusual men? Yes, and there are many other unusual men and women, most of them unknown, who live without self-pity, bitterness, or hostility and have no sense of stigma merely because they do not hear.

A SENSE OF COMMUNITY

Meeting at Gallaudet, a college for prelingually deaf people, and a large, bustling, vibrant, mainly young community where hearing persons may feel like interlopers—seminar members often discussed the differences between those who are deafened early versus late in life, between the deaf who grow old and the old who grow deaf. The differences, not similarities, were stressed, and most comparisons tended to favor the prelingually deaf.

Those deafened early have many handicaps: difficulty in learning to speak, voices that sound strange and may be hard to understand, educational retardation, and a limited choice of professions and occupations with limited prospects for advancement. They face the difficulties and dangers to which all who cannot hear are exposed in a world organized principally by and for the hearing, a world through which they pass in isolated groups, like visiting foreigners.

Yet, never having heard, they experience no struggle between remaining in or withdrawing from hearing society. They often have deaf family members and friends, attend schools for the deaf, and have a deaf spouse and children: in short, they have comfortable companionship. In contrast, hard-of-hearing adults usually have a hearing family, spouse, children, and friends, who, showing greater or lesser patience and sympathy, are often at the center of their discomfort. With a language of their own, prelingually deaf persons enjoy easy communication with fellow signers, escaping the anxiety about misunderstanding and missing speech that is a central aggravation for the hard of hearing. Their serious problems of communicating with nonsigners are practical, not emotional, like those of an American in Albania or a Swede in Tibet.

Above all, deaf persons have a culture and community of their own, which gives them a sense of identity, unity, and self-respect that permits them to persevere, to help one another, to relax, socialize, and enjoy life despite their injuries and misfortunes in hearing society. Schein (1968), Becker (1980), Higgins (1980), and Owens (1981), among others, have elaborated this picture of a deaf community. It has theoretical roots in and descriptive parallels with anthropological studies of peasant and modern communities, the work of Chicago sociologists, and the descriptions of neighborhood groups by Whyte (1943), Gans (1962), or Liebow (1967).

In contrast, hard-of-hearing persons are strikingly isolated, clinging to but cut off from the hearing community and with no distinctive language or culture of their own. Those who are well off can equip their homes with special phones, TDDs, audio loops, captioned TV, signal lights, and other devices. Where and how can they find a circle, a community where their hearing trouble is taken for granted, not unexpected and embarrassing? Can and should they form a community of their own?

In a passage cited by Meadow-Orlans (see p. 52), Kyle and Wood (1983) say that they do not want to form such communities:

> ... there is little desire to be part of a community of hard of hearing people in those who become deaf. The idea that those with handicaps might benefit from personal contact with other people with the same problem is not considered to be of much relevance. In practice, it is just as easy to lipread or hear a hearing person as it is to have contact with someone else with acquired deafness.

That is most true of persons with a moderate hearing loss, whom Kyle and his colleagues have studied, and is doubtlessly also true of many, but certainly not all, with a severe hearing loss. The existence of Self Help for Hard of Hearing People (SHHH), Washington Area Group for the Hard of Hearing (WAGHOH), Consumers Organization for the Hearing Impaired (COHI), and Organization for the Use of the Telephone (OUT), numerous speech and hearing societies, church groups, and other formal and informal local groups organized by and for hearing-impaired people demonstrates that.

Some clarification of the concept of "community" and its applicability to the prelingually and adventitiously deafened populations may be useful.

In its traditional usage in the anthropological and sociological literature, a community consisted of the residents of a compact area, typically a town or village or perhaps a rural township or parish, who knew one another, shared common experiences, and were linked by economic and social activities, family and friendship, and shared culture and moral values. The concept was more than a little romantic; the idea of "community" as a place of brotherhood and peace evoked Rousseau's idyll of man in a state of nature.

Clearly, in referring to the prelingually deaf community, the elements of economic interdependence and physical proximity can be attenuated, although the physical proximity is found in residential schools, at Gallaudet College, and the Columbus Colony housing project in Westerville, Ohio. The emphasis is primarily on common characteristics, experience, language, type of education, needs, interests, self-identification, and ready identifiability, although community members are scattered in thousands of places across the nation.

Albert Pimentel challenged the simplistic notion of a single unified "deaf community." A community, he observed, is multifaceted and dynamic. To "mainstream" deaf children in hearing schools weakens the deaf community. Captioned films once brought deaf people together; captioned TV now separates them. The "deaf community" is fragmented into many groups with special interests. Fringe groups derive satisfaction from it; gay, old, young, or professional people may enter and leave. And adventitiously deafened persons who stand aloof may benefit from some of its services, such as the provision of information on hearing loss and hearing aids.

Not all members of the "deaf community" are prelingually deaf, as is apparent from their clear and natural speech. Some became deaf in their teens and others, later in life. It would be instructive to learn why this small fraction of people deafened in adulthood have identified with the deaf when the majority regard signing as a worse stigma than a hearing aid. As Howard Stone remarked, the hard of hearing harbor the same prejudice against the deaf as hearing people do. Some, profoundly deafened for years, after failing to maintain their hearing friends, come to appreciate the virtues of signing.

The overwhelming majority of hard of hearing and deafened adults want little or nothing to do with the deaf. In any event, they cannot sign, so how can they communicate? They see not the admirable strengths of the deaf community but instead may think *these people are stone deaf, God spare me their condition*. Indeed, as Kyle and Wood observed, most hard of hearing adults probably also want little or nothing to do with other hard of hearing people; they want to continue with their old friends, not pick a new set with similar hearing troubles. But these feelings can change as their hearing worsens and their friends, or they themselves, find their efforts at conversation too frustrating.

Once it emerges, a sense of community with other deafened persons can be sustained by very little. Lonely, elderly people, cut off from human contact by retirement, deafness, and timidity, can derive comfort from a handwritten note from a SHHH volunteer, from reading the bimonthly *Shhh* journal, even from writing about their experiences and feelings in response to a questionnaire on hearing loss. Most do not attend the local meetings or national conventions: they are too feeble or poor, live too far away, have lost the habit of socializing, or have almost as much trouble conversing with a patient hard-of-hearing person as with an impatient hearing one. Nonetheless, SHHH and its journal mean a great deal to them: it means that they are not alone.

A long list of practical measures that would help hard of hearing people can be compiled. If SHHH grew tenfold or found a wealthy patron or if an effective federation of professional and voluntary associations concerned with deafness were formed, most could be undertaken readily. The Oyers present one such list (see p. 151). I would stress a service to provide information on the quality, reliability, and cost of different hearing aids and assistive devices; audiological diagnosis and prescription that is independent of the distribution of particular brands; reimbursement for audiological services and hearing aids in medical insurance; research to improve aids, especially by filtering background noise and making the volume control more convenient; and a service to install audio loops and other devices.

The repertoire of rehabilitation programs should be augmented by research and instruction on the practical problems that hearing people, both novices and those with extensive experience, face in dealing with the hard of hearing. To ascribe to stigma and ignorance all the difficulties the hard of hearing encounter with the hearing is unjust and simplistic. The lipreader is not the only one who can be fatigued; when time is short, as it is on many occasions in a normal day, explanations must be cut short; the novice, who is nonplussed—not scornful—needs immediate guidance. The hard of hearing and the hearing will get on better when they understand each other better; each pair (spouses, friends, or acquaintances) must jointly reach the distinctive accommodation that best suits their joint needs.

The advantages of a residential community for hard-of-hearing people will be known better after one has been established. It should not and cannot be confined to the hearing impaired who, after all, have hearing families and friends. All that is needed is a critical density—10 or 20 per cent in a given area should suffice.

From such a concentration much would follow naturally to ease the life of hard-of-hearing residents. From notices, word of mouth, and repeated encounters, those living in or visiting the neighborhood would learn of its special character. Knowing that hard-of-hearing people live there, residents, shopkeepers, bank tellers, waiters, delivery and service people, policemen, firefighters, postal workers, and bus and cab drivers would expect to meet them and learn to communicate with them.

The heightened demand should often bring improved services and facilities. The neighborhood theater would show captioned films, the local churches and school auditorium would install audio loops, the library would carry a collection of books and periodicals on hearing loss and hearing services, the hospital dispatcher would alert ambulance crews to the hearing-impaired community. Information about hearing aids, clinics, assistive devices, captioned TV programs, and the like would be readily available. One neighbor might inspect and try out another's audio or visual equipment and learn where to get one. Community groups would work to improve the safety and comfort of residents—for example, by getting signs posted to alert drivers to the presence of deafened people, having suitable phones installed in public places and a TDD in the local police and fire stations. The absence of surprises and the expectation of informed and courteous service would make daily life easier and more relaxing.

A perceptive real estate company or a few hard-of-hearing friends could start such a community simply by buying homes or apartments near one another. The Swedish factory town cited by Meadow-Orlans (see p. 44) is one such community, and a group of steel workers in Wheeling, West Virginia, is another. However, both developed naturally as a result of progressive deafness in factory workers. Who will consciously form the first community of and for hearing-impaired persons?

IN CONCLUSION

This chapter started with the question, "Do numbers count?" The answer, at present, must be "no" or "not sufficiently." The very large number of persons whose hearing is impaired in adulthood has not received adequate attention from researchers, practitioners, service providers, those who develop and manufacture auditory equipment, and others able to advance their welfare. In part, this is due to the heterogeneity of the population, encompassing individuals whose degrees of hearing loss and ages vary greatly; to the variety of their interests and needs; and hence to their lack of common purpose and common action on their own behalf. The great majority of hearing-impaired people have preferred silent suffering to uniting to improve their lot.

However, there are signs—e.g., the formation of SHHH, the 1981 Mini-Conference on Elderly Hearing-Impaired People, and the 1980 and 1984 International Congresses for Hard of Hearing People in Hamburg and Stockholm—that this situation may be changing. Further examination of the needs of hearing-impaired persons and further measures to serve them are likely as their numbers grow with the growth of the elderly population.

Hearing aids and assistive devices, communal assistance, and encouragement can help someone with a hearing loss, if he or she wants the help. But, in the final analysis, the task of adjustment, of living with the disability, is up to the individual. Deafness can be a torment that makes life unbearable or merely, as Howard Stone put it, "another of life's trials." To a question about what enabled her to cope with her husband's deafness, Pauline Ashley replied with some exasperation, "He's still Jack Ashley. He's still the same person who just happens to have gone deaf. It was just a damn nuisance."

Two authors in this volume quote the same anguished passage of Beethoven's, but neither refers to the triumph of the Ninth Symphony or the late quartets. Martineau wrote that "deafness is about the best thing that ever happened to me;—the best, in a selfish view, as the grandest impulse to self-mastery" (1983, I, p. 78). Thomas Edison, whose hearing was impaired at the age of 12 and grew progressively worse thereafter, said that "my deafness has been not a handicap but a help to me." It drove him to reading and enabled him to concentrate without distraction. It helped him in business, leading him to avoid verbal agreements and to "have everything set down in black and white." He attributes his invention of the phonograph and the carbon transmitter, which made Alexander Graham Bell's telephone successful, to his deafness. And deafness helped his courtship. " . . . it excused me for getting quite a little nearer to her than I would [otherwise] have dared . . . . And after things were actually going nicely, I found hearing unnecessary."

It may be said that I was shut off from that particular kind of social intercourse which is small talk. I am glad of it . . . . I have no doubt that my nerves are stronger and better today than they would have been if I had heard all the foolish conversation and other meaningless sounds that normal people hear . . . .

People with good hearing have become so accustomed to the uproar of civilization that that uproar has become necessary to their lives. If all the noise suddenly would stop on Broadway, Broadwayites would faint away. Broadway as it is is a peaceful thoroughfare to me . . . .

We are building a world in which the person who is deaf will have a definite advantage. If we keep on as we are going we shall have a general environment which will be impossible to the acutely hearing person. (Edison, 1968, pp. 44-56)

Edison writes at such length, with such conviction and good humor, we dare not say his is a case of sour grapes. It appears that, with an unusual inventive talent and self-sufficient character, he not only overcame but exploited his deafness to achieve a greater measure of success than would otherwise have been probable. That fullest measure of adjustment may be rare, but it points to the direction others can follow. To accept one's condition and find fulfillment in it is the beginning and perhaps the end of wisdom.

REFERENCES

Allan, T., and Gordon, S. (1952). *The scalpel, the sword: The story of Norman Bethune*. Boston: Little, Brown.

Becker, G. (1980). *Growing old in silence*. Berkeley: University of California Press.

DiMichael, S. G. (1983, September/October). Assertiveness training for hard-of-hearing people. *Shhh, 4*(5), 3-5.

Edison, T. A., (Runes, D. D., ed.) (1968). *The diary and sundry observations of Thomas Alva Edison*. New York: Greenwood Press.

Gans, H. J. (1962). *The urban villagers*. New York: Free Press.

Goffman, E. (1963). *Stigma, notes on the management of spoiled identity*. Englewood Cliffs, NJ: Prentice-Hall.

Heider, F., and Heider, G. M. (1941). Studies in the psychology of the deaf, No. 2. *Psychological Monographs, 53*, 5 (Whole No. 242).

Higgins, P. C. (1980). *Outsiders in a hearing world*. Beverly Hills, CA: Sage.

Kyle, J. G., and Wood, P. L. (1983, April). *Social and vocational aspects of acquired hearing loss*. Final Report to MSC, School of Education Research Unit, University of Bristol, England.

Lehmann, R. R. (1954). Bilateral sudden deafness. *New York State Journal of Medicine, 54*, 1481-1484.

Liebow, E. (1967). *Tally's corner*. Boston: Little, Brown.

Martineau, H. (1983). *Autobiography*. London: Virago Press. (Two volumes, first published 1877.)

Orlans, H., and Meadow-Orlans, K. P. (1984). Who are the members of SHHH? A report on the *Shhh* questionnaire. *Shhh, 5*(5), 3-5.

Owens, D. J. (1981). *The relationship of frequency and types of activity to life satisfaction in elderly deaf people.* Unpublished doctoral dissertation, School of Education, Health and Nursing Arts, New York University.

Ries, P. W. (1982). *Hearing ability of persons by sociodemographic and health characteristics: United States* (Series 10, No. 140). National Center for Health Statistics. Washington, DC: U.S. Government Printing Office.

Schein, J. D. (1968). *The deaf community.* Washington, DC: Gallaudet College Press.

Singer, J. D., with Tomberlin, T. J., Smith, J. M., and Schrier, A. J. (1982, March). *Analysis of noise-related auditory and associated health problems in the U.S. adult population (1971-1975).* Prepared for Environmental Protection Agency, Washington, DC by Abt Associates, U.S. Department of Commerce National Technical Information Service, Vol. 1.

Whyte, W. F. (1943). *Street corner society.* Chicago: University of Chicago Press.

Author Index

Subject Index

Page numbers in *italics* refer to illustrations, (t) indicates a table.

A

C

D